ARE
YOU
REALLY
THE
DOCTOR?

ARE YOU REALLY THE DOCTOR?

MY LIFE AS A BLACK DOCTOR IN THE NHS

Matthew Hutchinson

First published in the UK in 2025 by Blink Publishing
An imprint of Bonnier Books UK
5th Floor, HYLO, 105 Bunhill Row,
London, EC1Y 8LZ

A CIP catalogue record for this book is available from the British Library.

Hardback ISBN: 9781785121340

Also available as an ebook and an audiobook

1 3 5 7 9 10 8 6 4 2

Design and Typeset by Envy Design Ltd
Printed and bound in Great Britain by Clays Ltd, Elcograf S.p.A.

The authorised representative in the EEA is
Bonnier Books UK (Ireland) Limited.
Registered office address: Floor 3, Block 3, Miesian Plaza,
Dublin 2, D02 Y754, Ireland
compliance@bonnierbooks.ie

www.bonnierbooks.co.uk

Dedicated to my parents, my wife and our children.

In memory of Alphonso Hutchinson.

CONTENTS

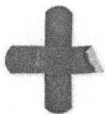

Prologue

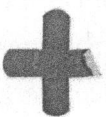

'WHO ARE YOU THEN!?'

'Like I said, I'm one of the doctors on the medical team.'

'Oh yeah? And what do you want?'

'I need to ask you a few questions, see how you're doing.'

'Christ, can't you just leave me alone? It's three in the morning.'

This from a 22-year-old man who had staggered into A&E after a night out. The tone of his Yorkshire accent was angry and abrasive, as opposed to the gentle, broadband-flogging aural comfort blanket that TV adverts have made us soft southern folk accustomed to.

As tempting as it would be to oblige at this point and have a break instead, duty and my (possibly misguided) desire to hang on to my licence to practice meant I was forced to plough on.

'You told the A&E doctors you had a headache, and it was really bad?'

'You're telling me.'

'Was it the worst headache you've ever had?'

'Let me put it this way, I thought someone had come up and hit me on the head from behind with a hammer.'

He looked at me in a way that suggested he thought I wasn't man enough to recognise a hammer if it hit me, and was then dangled up in front of my face.

My heart sank. He was saying all of the right things to create both worry and work. Headaches are, quite frankly, despite the name, a pain in the arse. Most of the cases you end up seeing are benign, but given the organ involved, the ones that aren't have a nasty habit of being life-threatening. Once the Emergency Department team refer a severe 'thunderclap' headache, the wheels are set in motion. It could be nothing, but in around 20 per cent of cases it's the sign that a murderous little berry aneurysm in a blood vessel has ripened and decided to burst, decanting claret into your skull, and leaving your brain dangerously cramped, squashed against the bone.

It meant we were going to have to unsheathe a long, threatening needle, pierce between the bones of his spine and take a sample from the fluid that bathes the cord and brain, to check for evidence of bleeding.

'And I understand you had been at the pub?'

Already a picture of annoyance, his face contorted further.

'Look, this isn't because of drink – I know what I can drink. I'd had about five pints. Hardly a skinful.'

'No, sure . . . but it's all important.'

The fact he considered five pints a quiet Thursday evening drink was probably a clue as to why he wasn't a picture of robust health. I trudged on a little further, trying to get the rest of the history, looking in vain for an offramp, but in reality, the path had already been set.

I made it through just about enough of a neurological examination (the 'touch your nose, follow my finger' routine that makes you feel like you're on a hidden camera show) to satisfy myself his brain wasn't about to squeeze through the escape hatch in the base of his skull, before he completely ran out of patience.

'Look, just piss off and let me sleep.'

I could definitely leave him alone for now, but whether he would get any sleep was another matter, given the hourly neurological observations he'd be getting.

* * *

By the time the morning post-take ward round (the consultant, trailed by underlings, tasked with reviewing the night team's work) reached him, a night of regular waking to have a torch shone in his eyes had sweetened him even further.

'Dr Hutchinson tells me you had a severe headache?'

'Yes . . . and can I say I thought he looked scruffy.'

Dr Simmons was evidently taken aback by this additional titbit of information. Attempting to remain jovial, he offered:

'I don't see what's wrong with what he's wearing.'

'No, very scruffy . . . you sure he's trained?'

Much of the reason he and everyone else on the post-take medical team looked perplexed, and more than a little uncomfortable, likely stemmed from the fact that I was wearing scrubs, the pyjama-like, hospital-issue uniform – something that it's pretty difficult to put your own personal flair on, scruffy or otherwise. This left only a few things he could be objecting to: skin, hair or general . . . 'vibe'.

Dr Simmons became noticeably stern at this point. 'Well I *don't* agree. And yes, having made it onto this specialty *training* programme, I can assure you he's very well trained.'

A tall balding white man in his fifties, the kindly (by the bilious standards of many of his consultant colleagues) Dr Simmons was a respiratory physician by trade, peering inside smoke-blackened lungs, and thus used to dealing with whatever patients coughed up and spat his way with a smile. Ever supportive of his juniors, however, he had his limits.

'Anyway, this isn't what we need to be talking about. From the history, I'm worried you've had a bleed into your brain – perhaps damaging the area responsible for manners, and we need to know for sure. We're going to do a test called a lumbar puncture.'

It's always refreshing witnessing Caucasian seniority and impunity wielded in the name of good. He proceeded to list the reasoning and risks in as perfunctory and unempathetic a manner as he could muster and, once completed, turned and swept the ward round out of the room.

'I was reading . . . a CT angiogram is as good as an LP for detecting a subarachnoid, without being invasive,' I offered – still possessed of a puppy-like eagerness to demonstrate to the boss that I knew how to read, and was using these skills for the good of my ongoing medical education.

Dr Simmons permitted what I could have sworn was a half smile, and an almost conspiratorial look. 'Well, it's a shame we *don't* have the facility to do that sort of scan – and that nice man will have to have a painful procedure instead.'

* * *

Responses like this from patients, although not necessarily every day, are something staff from minority ethnic (global majority) groups in the NHS know to prepare themselves for. Patients have the same mix of virtue vying with terrible opinions as wider society, which, coupled with the small stress of a brush with mortality, means that along with the bodily fluids, the worst is likely to spill out at some point.

The mirror of this is that the people working in healthcare, and the structures they build, are influenced by the best and worst of our nature (though hopefully more of the former). This shapes the experience of these same ethnic groups as they access services and navigate the system.

I have been a doctor since 2012, and although I now specialise in rheumatology, acute general medicine remains a core part of the job. It is a quirk of the UK system that a lot of the work done by internists (generalists) in other countries is still done by specialists in respiratory (lungs – see above), gastroenterology (guts), and renal (kidneys) medicine – and, yes, rheumatology (we'll come to that).

I have the utmost respect for my colleagues for whom acute medicine is their one true calling – becoming expert in sifting and managing the unsorted wash of medical patients (the ones the surgeons can't help by chopping bits out/off of them) coming into the hospital, comfortable with any cardiac arrhythmia, and happy to ram large needles into any central vein or chest cavity.

I have equal respect for those specialised doctors who have chosen to forgo the churn and chaos of general medicine, to focus on the specific thing they do best. Many of my most expert mentors have done just that. But there is a romantic part of me that clings to the idea that medicine in A&E and the admissions unit is a noble tradition, a grindstone that helps keep specialists sharp and in touch with the wider hospital.

Then there is the other half of my job. Becoming a rheumatologist requires a certain amount of humility. Seriously, I am the Michael Jordan of modesty. As much as I am secure in my belief that what we do is valuable, it is a little difficult to be too arrogant when 99 per cent of people have no idea what you do – or think it mainly involves oiling and massaging the creaking joints of the elderly (not to downplay the importance of this). Every blank look when you tell people your speciality is another serving of that ego-choking humble pie.

'Is that bones?'

'Sure, sometimes, yes – more joints – but it's so much *more* than that . . .'

You can hear the pleading in my voice as I try to explain that although it started out as the non-surgical treatment of musculoskeletal disease, we see a range of exciting things and now have (often expensive) drugs that actually work.

Broadly speaking, these days our remit is inflammatory diseases caused by a misbehaving immune system – usually affecting the joints, true, but also often attacking many other organs in the body. Rheumatoid arthritis is our bread and butter, an autoimmune disease that, despite misconceptions, can strike at any age and affects around 1 per cent of the population. If not treated properly, it can lead to severe disability, an invisible force irreversibly twisting limbs and digits.

Lupus, another favourite, *does* also cause arthritis, but the inflammation can cause damage anywhere – a situation that for obvious reasons can quickly become life-threatening, when white blood cells start chewing away at kidneys, lungs or heart.

It's still not really dinner party medicine on a par with surgery or cardiology though, is it? Tales of antibodies and autoimmunity hardly leave companions swooning over their starters at your sweaty-browed heroism.

Almost all of our conditions cause chronic pain, and often fatigue that is even worse. These can be intractable, even when the inflammation is gone. In a cycle of mutual feeding, these diseases make already hard lives harder, and are themselves made heavier burdens by poor housing, working conditions and caring responsibilities.

This may perhaps all seem a little niche, special interest – but lupus disproportionately affects non-white patients, and they fare less well. The disease is poorly understood, meaning there is often a delay in diagnosis, since doctors often don't recognise rashes they've only seen in textbooks on white skin, or don't take seriously the non-specific symptoms they chalk up to 'ethnic quirkiness and manifestations of stress'. The experiences of these lupus patients are some of the most crystalline examples of how the NHS treats migrants and their descendants.

With this book, I'll explore the impact of race on healthcare in the NHS – both the experiences of non-white staff, how they are treated and the contribution they make. Despite being integral to the establishment of the health service, and forming the backbone of many staff groups (39 per cent of nursing staff are from non-white ethnic groups), they face discrimination and remain underrepresented in senior positions. These doctors, nurses and midwives are more likely to face professional sanctions, in particular those educated abroad.

The expression 'trust me, I'm a doctor' comes a lot less easily if you have to spend extra energy even convincing the indignant patient in front of you that you are one. Many people still have a fixed picture of what a doctor looks like (i.e., a middle-aged white guy). Take, for example, the response to the announcement of a black Doctor Who. If some members of the public can't cope with a time-travelling, shape-shifting alien being black, you can bet they probably have similar thoughts when it comes to brain surgeons.

I'll explore the structures and traditions that are in place and serve as obstacles to progress within healthcare professions. Starting at university, this can be the Latin you didn't learn at state school cropping up in medical terminology to confuse you, and the language and accent you *do* use marking you out as different.

I'll also discuss what accessing the NHS is like for patients from minority backgrounds. For some (but by no means all), a trip to the doctor is a visit to see someone they might rarely encounter socially – a privileged representative of the establishment. The effect of this on agency and the ability to advocate shouldn't be underestimated. Nor can we overlook the (hopefully) unconscious effect that struggling to relate to the patient in front of them can have on the efforts of healthcare staff and the care they receive.

These factors feed into measurably worse outcomes for black and other non-white patients, across all areas of medicine. Black women are four times more likely to die during childbirth. Black people are eight times more likely to be admitted to hospital with lupus. Mental health outcomes are no better. Black people are almost five times as likely to be detained under the Mental Health Act, and ten times more likely to be subject to a community treatment order.

All of this may sound a little heavy-going – and it can be. Away from the hospital, I work as a comedian – something I will bring to these stories. ('A spoon full of sugar' or 'laughter is the best medicine' – pick your cliche.) Comedy can help us cope with the harsh realities in these stories, without forgetting that the patients at the heart of them is what really matters. Hopefully, my colleagues can take a joke, and forgive me for any well-meaning ribbing (sorry, cardiology, I love you really!).

* * *

The evening after a run of nights is a jet-lagged limbo, the first taste of freedom muted, not fully present. Friday in the park, there is a low, euphoric buzz. Impromptu picnic groups on the hill beam and clink plastic wine tumblers, the Weekend supplement idyll of August fun. The light of the day's end stains the sky with a citrus blush, the polluted alchemy of London's smog, the metalwork teeth of the city in the northern distance softened by the haze.

Ending an afternoon of furtive attempts to strike up small talk with fellow parents in the playground, millennial Radio 6 Music dads coax their kids down from the swings come home time. This is south London's answer to Primrose Hill – although marginally less crowded when the sun's out – and no, I won't tell you where it is. It wasn't always like this. It is the same park some friends were afraid to come and hang out in as teenagers, fearing the very real prospect of being robbed, or worse.

In my daze I watch the aerial display transfixed. They dive low over the long dry grass, the patch of the field left to grow, then scorch in the late-summer sun that will soon be dipping below the horizon. With their wings tucked, at first glance they could be mistaken for starlings in close formation – at least by someone with my limited understanding of the outdoors. (A childhood dedicated to indoor screen pursuits in darkened rooms didn't provide much opportunity for birdwatching.)

Looking for any length of time, the plumage offers quick correction – the unmistakable vibrant lime green of parakeets. That and the noise. To our ears it may not register as birdsong, but the warbling, clucking chirp is now the constant soundtrack to an early evening in the park, injecting energy and life.

There is a great deal of folklore regarding the origin of these birds, how London became host to these tropical interlopers. Did they escape a film set? Did Jimi Hendrix set them free? Or is their presence the result of many years of displacement through captivity, followed by release, thriving against the odds in an alien and supposedly inhospitable environment? Whatever the truth, one thing is certain: they didn't fly here themselves (I googled it, they don't migrate).

We are in Lewisham, which has always been one of the more deprived London boroughs. As a whole, it still is, but an increasing number of bubbles have formed, sustaining organic markets, craft ale bottle shops and purveyors of eye-wateringly expensive antipasti bobbing seductively in jars of olive oil.

This is where my parents have lived for all my life – and now, for me, social mobility has simply meant being able to afford to stay put. It's a measure of both the unrelenting march of gentrification and the cost of simply being alive, that affording to buy a three-bedroom house in Catford is enough to mark you out as bourgeois scum. I say this not to garner any sympathy, but when this is a stretch for two doctors in their late thirties (if any casting directors are reading, my playing age remains 25–35) to afford, a profound change has happened. What hope is there for families on the average income, or less, to get by?

You can choose how you tell a story. I could be the son of an immigrant (my father came to the UK in the 1960s as a member of the Windrush generation) who made it from the mean streets of Lewisham to medical school. That *Fresh Prince of Bel Air* fantasy would certainly be an easy sell and, in the loosest sense, true, but it would contain a bigger lie. You'd be missing out the fact that my parents owned the house we lived in, that they were able to coach me into a nice secondary school in the suburbs, and that my father was a research scientist at the university I would ultimately attend. These privileges are no doubt the difference that has given me access to a career denied to many others who were similarly able.

It would be absurd for me to emulate so many authors writing from a secure vantage point, claiming some working-class origin story. But, equally, I have spent my life perched on the fence, not distant from either side of the social divide – undoubtedly feeding my world view and attracting the fatal accusation of centrism.

I grew up in a perfectly nice semi-detached house, but in a postcode that would raise a concerned eyebrow. That we were actually on a hill just outside of, and overlooking, this supposedly scary place was apparently beside the point for many people when I told them where I lived. At home, we were about as educationally privileged as it is possible to be. Both my parents have PhDs, although, I hate to break it to you, they don't tend to pay post-doctoral scientists the big bucks (medium bucks at best). This mismatch between financial reward and workload, coupled with the job insecurity, was a major factor in them nudging me away from science and into medicine.

Now, if you ever hear me complaining publicly about my own experience of the cost of living, feel free to remind me that my wife owns a horse. Not that I have any say in the matter of course. A useful shorthand to convey the very worst upper-crust excesses, this fits a pair of cement shoes and throws overboard any 'man of the people' credentials I might aspire to. (In case you're wondering, the monthly cost is roughly the same as that more modern signifier of out-of-touch douchery – the lease on an entry-level Tesla.)

There is of course the obvious, 50 per cent white elephant in the room. That is, my dual heritage. I grew up 'mixed race', trained to correct anyone who dared use the dreaded 'half caste', only for my own terminology, in turn, to become faux pas. It is a strange, destabilising feature of belonging to a minoritised group, to be classified according to some external criteria, make your peace with it, only to later find you need to sign up to the updated racial terms and conditions.

For some, this may be enough to disqualify me from even writing this book. To them, my blackness would at best be probationary; the black card I was issued only provisional. In his book *Natives*, Akala employs the term 'racialised as black' with devastating clarity – highlighting that in white-dominated Western societies, people with appreciable African ancestry have historically and continue to be classified as black, a widely pervasive 'One Drop' philosophy that was in the past even enshrined in law in the US. It would be unwise to ever forget this. I will refer to myself and family members using both the terms 'black' and 'dual heritage'.

Even so, I can't ignore the impact of class, colourism, nationality, language and accent on experience. These factors all impact acceptance and opportunity, and I hold up my light-skinned, uncallused hands to the fact that I have benefited.

I wouldn't be so unwise as to claim to speak for all people; I can only tell stories as I have experienced and observed them. There will also be stories of interactions with members of other minoritised groups, which, although important to include, are no substitute for hearing from them first hand.

Not everything I describe will be typical, because I don't think that's possible. There seems to be a temptation to cast black life in the UK as all struggle, or alternatively to pretend we now live and work within enlightened structures, watched over by our diversity and inclusion guardian angels.

The stories told here are all true, at least in the way memories are true. All recall is the eternally redrafted artist's impression, with highlights, smears and touch-ups guided by emotion and self-image.

For the avoidance of doubt, however, I'll be clear that some specifics have been changed. For the most part, this is the editing of demographic and at times medical case details to avoid patients being recognisable.

The details of medical staff and the hospitals have again been altered and left deliberately vague. I am all for speaking truth to power, however I certainly don't have the reserves for a libel case, even when the events in question definitely happened.

A few timelines have also been compressed for the sake of brevity, since neither you nor I want this book to be double the length in the name of painstaking chronological accuracy. Please do forgive me.

CHAPTER 1

In a Strange Land (Called Essex)

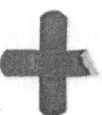

IN ONE OF my more unimaginative teenage moments, I decided my 18th birthday should coincide with another rite of passage – going on a 'lads' holiday (or the closest to that I could bear). Happy to just be involved, I signed on unquestioningly to a weekend of rain- and beer-soaked camping in Newquay. This was despite already being firmly of the opinion that sleeping in a tent is an activity that should be reserved for when something has gone seriously wrong in life – natural disaster, war, or, at a push, attending a music festival.

Among the group were my good friends Joel and Ruari, along with some more vague acquaintances whose defining shared characteristic was that they were massive stoners (if the GMC are reading, I'm certainly *not* including myself in that description – the wackiest thing you'll find in my house is a bottle of natural wine I'm pretending to enjoy a little more than I really do). Envisage the laziest teen movie depiction of a group of slackers, and you won't be far off. The budget approach permeated every element, so I found myself bundled onto the National Express, the air thick with badinage, fuelled by energy drinks and surrounded by only semi-ironically purchased lads' mags.

'The doctor's doing his "research"' was the cry as the contents of the WH Smith's carrier bag containing the coach trip's entertainment was assessed.

Arriving at the campsite, we were stricken by a procession of issues – first, it was at least a mile's walk from town. Second, the holiday season wasn't in full swing yet – meaning everything was much quieter than we had banked on. Third – none of us surfed, so there was very little, if anything, to actually do during the day – other than sit and ruminate on why we weren't in Spain.

The starting pistol for a weekend of fun was fired by a gathering around three disposable barbecues, prodding at limp grey burgers with improvised utensils – half a pair of wooden tongs and a rusty bread knife. Our collective adolescent cooking skills allowed us to somehow dodge the inevitable bullet of food poisoning – a prospect too grim to consider in the strained toilet facilities on a sodden campsite.

Buoyed by our culinary success, we headed into Newquay. I'd be lying if I said I can accurately recall the logic that led to us drinking on the streets by the seafront, but it likely involved some reverse snobbery – we didn't want to spend money we didn't have in bars we had already decided were full of arseholes. Plus, al fresco drinking is what we would have been doing back home anyway, so why break the habit?

Adventurously, and arguably unwisely, we had climbed over the waist-high metal railing and perched on a cliff edge above the beach. By our standards, this was a pretty civilised way of passing the time – waves lapping, backlit by the town around the bay.

After half an hour or so, we became aware of four locals standing and staring. They were just the other side of the railing, blocking the path between us and safety. In sportswear and polo shirts, they were what curtain twitchers might describe as 'youths' up to no good. In pure cinematic cliche, the shortest, skinniest among them was the one with the mouth:

'What are you doing here, dark horse?'

Perhaps caught off guard by this injection of diversity to the town, he had grasped for a phrase both racially offensive and threatening, but found something that, if anything, just ended up confusing. Still, the intent was clear – and we faced the prospect of being hurled down the rock face by cider-soaked louts.

They didn't seem keen to cross the barrier, however. Perhaps even through the veil of White Lightning, they could see that a wrestling match on the precipice posed as much risk to them as it did to us. So we maintained a stalemate for what may have only been seconds, but felt an age – only broken when one of the stoners, Oli, showed an uncharacteristic spark of initiative, or pure self-interested cowardice, depending on your perspective. Possessed by a sudden mountain goat spirit, he descended to the beach below and loped across the sand and out of sight.

The threat in the faces of our tormenters turned to concern.

'Where's he going, to get your boys?'

What led them to the assumption that we had some yet unseen 'boys' as backup, contactable only by sprinting foot messenger, I'll never know, but it was too good an opportunity to pass up. We went with it.

'Yeah, he has . . . they'll be here soon . . .' Ruari managed to improvise, or simply agree, out of fear.

'Yeah, loads of them,' Joel added, perhaps overdoing it.

This seemed to have the desired effect. Their bonfire had been pissed on, and desire to fight dampened. They muttered noncommittally among themselves, and through half-audible grunts clearly decided there may be easier, less reinforced pickings elsewhere.

Sticking out at times is an occupational hazard for anyone non-white in the UK – more frequent the more you hang out with white people, going to the places they drag you to. Eventually you learn where you're willing to brave in the name of fun – often a select group of major cities, nowhere too remote.

For similar reasons, having some say over where you live is important – being able to stay near a community you recognise, where you might be able to blend in. I for one am not in a rush to move to Chatham, or Ipswich, or Durham.

The first two years out of medical school are composed of the 'foundation programme' – four-month rotational jobs in a mix of specialties, some you'll inevitably be more interested in than others. Until recently, in the final year of medical school, students participated in a brutal trial that would determine where they worked and therefore lived. They sat the 'situational judgement test' – designed to make sure you will be a safe doctor, but filled with asinine questions:

'You are working on a busy ward, and notice your consultant comes in to work smelling of alcohol. Do you:

A – High-five him for being a bloody good lad

B – Ask for a swig

C – Slap him around the face and demand his badge and his gun (stethoscope), because he's in no fit state

D – Excuse yourself and seek help from a senior colleague, as your consultant is currently posing a danger to patients'

Your score in this test was then combined with your ranking among your peers (at your university only) from end-of-year exams, and, based on this, the machine might spit you out anywhere from Brighton to Aberdeen. I have nothing against Aberdeen. I have actually never been there, which I think is also pretty good grounds for not being forced to live somewhere.

The spectre of job applications menaced any student from the very beginning of university. In my time, whispers descended from the years above about the best ways to avoid banishment. There was a rumour that being social secretary of a sports team gained you more points on the application than being able to remember the bones in the wrist, and so people with no prior interest in the sport suddenly found themselves, bleary-eyed and frost-bitten, braving the goose shit and rowing on the Thames at dawn.

As well as avoiding places they might not be familiar with, many soon-to-be doctors are also likely to avoid areas of major deprivation if given the choice, where the hospitals may be over-whelmed, the surroundings less genteel. An effect of this system could have been to send a cohort of lower-ranked, possibly less motivated recruits to areas of greatest need – although in reality, the reasons for less stellar academic performance will be varied, and impacted by social and economic factors, and I don't believe these graduates are necessarily any less capable of doing the job.

Anyway, this process has been replaced by something arguably worse: a lottery. Now, there is no way of even working hard to protect yourself. Instead, preferences are listed, and then life is decided on the basis of a glorified tombola. Your rank, and therefore order of choice, is decided at random.

This new system, although perhaps on the surface fairer on the patients and the hospitals, has proven almost universally unpopular. In the final year of their degree, after five and a half years of believing that hard work and a little extra revision would allow students to wrestle some control over their destiny, it arrived like the unwelcome surprise of a contact tracing call from the sexual health clinic. Students of this cohort describe feeling powerless, subject to the whims of the uncaring Mount Olympus of NHS management.

To non-white students, there is an additional set of fears associated with their destination – what type of racists do they have there? Prejudice and isolation are things that can be encountered in many places, but at least in Bermondsey or Mayfair I know what flavours I'm likely to get, generally. I know where I can and can't go. Scunthorpe, on the other hand – I'm not sure how they do things up there.

New medics from England have been sent unwillingly as far afield as Northern Ireland – another part of the UK I'm sure has plenty going for it, if that's where you want to be. But it is also one of the places that saw the most enthusiastic anti-immigration rioting during the unrest of August 2024. The UK non-white population is 18 per cent. In London, it's 46 per cent. Northern Ireland? 3.45 per cent.

In that position, asked to swap familiar multiculturalism for the prospect of rain and racism, I'd be inclined to tell the foundation programme to stick their job and quit – perhaps join the ranks of the graduate management consultants with no real-world work experience, but generous expense accounts. And that's what you would have to do, because, at the start of our careers, the NHS is a monopoly employer. You either take the only job you're offered, or you don't become a doctor.

By now, you might be keen to point out that many other jobs mean relocating, often with little say in where. But this isn't what we signed up for. We didn't join the army. I am also making myself ripe for the accusation of sounding like that most heinous villain – the liberal metropolitan elite, wanting to remain sheltered behind the walls of the city, hiding from the 'Real Britain'. While this may be somewhat true, it's driven by a desire to be somewhere I feel comfortable, and safe.

At six years long, medical school feels like it will last for ever, until all of a sudden it's done, and you're sitting in the launch seat, pointed at a new horizon. There is a strange limbo, after the moment of relief of opening the finals results email – being tempted and entitled to add 'Dr' to every last one of your accounts in the hope it might lend some gravitas to your next customer service showdown – but before you've actually done any actual doctoring. A sense of fraudulence mixed with the anxiety I felt about moving, about the work.

In the end, Essex was where I landed for my first year. Or, more specifically, a town that seemed committed to living up to many of the county's cliches. This wasn't a punishment, not an exile, just a function of the 'one in, one out' rule. To keep things balanced, if you wanted to do one year of Foundation in London, the other had to be somewhere a little less cosmopolitan.

I wasn't alone; half of the hospital's new intake came from our medical school. Like an extension of student life, we lived together – only with the unfamiliar twist that, being outside London, we could actually afford somewhere habitable, nice even. Ours had been a family home, a slice of new-build suburban dream fodder, left vacant thanks to a messy divorce, which our emotionally labile, filterless landlady was desperate to offload about at any opportunity, oversharing at every visit.

'I may be single and nearly fifty – but I'm still fuckable!'

I have replayed this conversation between Dave and Lianne a thousand times in my head – and I assure you, there is no socially acceptable way to respond when someone with the power to evict you says this mid-conversation.

'Have you tried . . . Tinder? There's divorcees on there too?' (The app had just come out, and finding love online was evolving into something more than just the preserve of creeps and losers.)

Dave struggling for words was out of character. He has the ease of someone for whom life seems to just work out. At university, he was the only person in our halls who landed a double room, when others were sharing. He would later go on to charm his way through the interview into the most sought-after surgical training job in London, only to decide medicine wasn't for him and sidestep into the real dream: a lucrative job in tech.

Along with Dave, I lived with Nimal – perpetually upbeat, if slightly eccentric and innocent. He drove his Audi hatchback wearing a pair of black gloves, like some boy racer assassin, because he was allergic to the steering wheel – just touching it brought him out in hives. I, on the other hand, am not a car guy, but the lack of public transport forced my hand. I became the proud owner of a ten-year-old Corsa that leaked when it rained. This was only partially remedied by my mother's suggestion of stuffing the footwells with nappies.

The hospital was a utilitarian tower squatting on a wasteland on the edge of town. Like almost any district general hospital you'd care to mention in the UK, it was overfull and understaffed. This is a norm we blindly accept – that the doctors in the provinces can safely look after twice as many patients as their tertiary teaching hospital counterparts, with more limited access to scans and treatments. You may struggle to get them to admit it, but ask most doctors where they'd go if they were seriously ill, and I'd be willing to bet that, on balance, most would skip the 'good enough' place nearby in favour of the gleaming academic centre of excellence, for the resources alone. This of course isn't a guarantee – some of the most headline-grabbing tragedies and travesties have come out of these places, and inflated egos can lead to airship-scale disasters.

Despite all the time spent on the wards, for the most part, medical school teaches you medicine, not the job of actually being a doctor. These are categorically not the same thing. You might in theory know the scan your patient needs, but if you don't know where to drop off the handwritten request card (still the system at this hospital back in 2012), or whom to plead with to actually make it happen, you, and by extension your patient, are fresh out of luck. To remedy this, the new offerings spend the week before they start for real 'shadowing' the outgoing cohort. They are new foals, tottering after gnarled old war horses who have seen too much over the course of a year on the wards.

The bottom of the pyramid in medicine is the foundation year one (FY1) doctor, or 'house officer'. On the ward round, the job is pretty self-explanatory – a scribe/personal assistant hybrid, tasked with recording the patient's problems, the consultant or registrar's assessment and learned opinion, and, arguably most importantly, the list of tasks that awaits you. The worst mistake you're likely to commit is failing to whisk the curtain across with a magicianly flourish fast enough for the boss's liking.

There is a strange chasm between this often-mindless work and what is expected of you when a patient starts trying to die and there aren't any grown-ups around. You're suddenly expected to be able to distinguish whether the writhing and grimacing is just trapped wind from the hospital's insulting microwave attempt at goulash, or because their abdomen's about to explode. In the grand old tradition of keeping it simple, when starting out, all of these situations are dealt with identically – using the alphabet. Fortuitously, the body systems happen to have been named in order of likelihood of killing you quickest:

'A: Airway – unobstructed and clear (evidence – he's screaming at me)

B: Breathing – definitely still breathing, quickly (evidence – ditto the above, he's managing to get enough air in to keep screaming at me)

C: Circulation – the bedsheets weren't this soaked and red this morning . . .'

In the knowledge that a couple of simulation sessions at medical school could never adequately prepare us for this sort of emergency, our wise elders, in whom we now had fanatical belief, gave a teaching session on what to actually do when called to do some life saving. This was complete with an explanation of how to write in the notes to prove we had done our job properly (writing down what you have done to justify yourself to an imagined court often seems to be as, if not more, important than doing it in medicine).

Patients were packed into every inch of the crumbling 1960s estate – a situation that only got worse in the winter. Overflow wards were created seemingly at random – medical teams would arrive at work only to find themselves responsible for patients bedded down in the cardiac cath lab waiting area, or newly opened 'modular buildings' (i.e. glorified prefab huts).

In hospitals, speciality teams are broadly split along the lines of surgery – basically high-stakes arts and craft and DIY, dedicated to cutting things out and sewing, stapling or bolting what's left back together (they assure me it's more complicated than that) – and medicine – where the focus is often on synthesising story, symptoms and vital signs into the justification for tinkering (often ineffectually) with the patient's drug chart.

Thankfully I started on urology, one of the surgical specialties, mainly plumbing focused on diagnosing and unblocking obstructions in the urinary tract. I was lucky, because this was the one team that was relatively well staffed, a situation that had arisen when one of the consultants had recently quit (so getting rid of any extra elective patients he would have brought in), and no one had been organised enough to take away his allocation of minions. To begin with, however, we were nowhere near good enough to take full advantage of the luxury of adequate and safe staffing. At best, it just allowed us to be ever so slightly less shambolic.

Our work mostly consisted of collecting the steady trickle of kidney stone patients admitted via the surgical take. Day after day of suddenly stricken, desperate and sweating individuals – wincing as they involuntarily tried to force tiny calcium razor blades from kidney to bladder. I say tiny, but these are often wider than the path – the delicate, sausage-casing-like ureter, which continually contracts to push them along in agonising peristaltic Mexican waves.

The round was led most days by Mr Aggarwal – a short Indian man with a chest like a fridge and a moustache like Tom Selleck. He was an 'associate specialist' in urology, a title that means different things in different places, but in his case meant a fully qualified urologist, on the specialist register, but whom it suited the hospital to keep from becoming a fully fledged consultant because he could be handed the less interesting surgeries and the undesired task of babysitting the junior doctors on the ward.

These vital team members are disproportionately overseas medical graduates. Up and down the UK, departments are propped up by experienced immigrant doctors like him, often sufficiently experienced to work as consultants, but held in limbo at a lower grade, with diminished pay and, in the eyes of some, standing.

One factor that might not have helped him was his temper –

which, thanks to our organisational shortcomings starting out, was tested almost constantly. Each round would begin so promisingly, so sweetly.

'Okay team.' He started each day calling us 'team' incessantly, as if the word alone would reassemble us after the previous day's explosions. 'Where do we start?'

What should have been the simple task of learning the names and locations of our new patients in fact involved chasing down the night doctors, who kept the hard copy of the surgical intake of patients. If we were lucky, they'd be in the office, where the patients were handed out and bartered. Inevitably, we wouldn't be ready when he arrived – even when Frida, our German colleague (valiantly upholding her country's reputation for efficiency), had come in before the rest of us to sort the list, in the vain hope that today would be the day we got it right.

'We've got two up here on SAU [the surgical assessment unit] – both have got stones confirmed on CT KUB [CT scan of the kidneys, ureters and bladder].'

This was good, not for the patient (kidney stones are agony, the type of pain men perhaps accurately, but unwisely, compare to childbirth, before being quickly bludgeoned by the death stare of any mothers in the room), but for us – something definitely urological that Mr A would get to fix by sticking a telescope into someone's urethra.

When we got down to the ward that housed a hodge-podge of mixed surgical patients, it all fell apart. Inevitably, the notes would have been scattered and we would have no idea who they were or what was wrong with them. Worse still was if someone had taken out the bladder irrigation catheter from a patient too soon, or there had been some other deviation. This would prompt a furious recitation of his mantra:

'How many times!? You make a plan, you stick to it!'

We had metamorphosised from his 'team' to wayward children. The worst would come if, as can happen, we found ourselves looking after a patient who should have been under another team – the peptic ulcer which he had correctly diagnosed as the real cause for the patient's dropping haemoglobin, as their colour faded, until their skin looked camouflaged among the sheets, or the inflammatory bowel disease flare that had somehow crept onto our list disguised as a stone.

'You tell the gastroenterology team to come here and take over their care!'

For some reason, gastroenterology seemed to attract a disproportionate amount of his rage. At the time, our priority as FY1s was ducking for cover, avoiding strays – but now his frustration is easier to understand, if not fully excuse. To spend each day overworked and underappreciated, when just trying to do the best for patients, will eventually get to you. And he really did care. He was hardly doing it for the glamour.

* * *

My start set the tone as far as the expectations of my friends and family were concerned. Parental pride soon turned to confusion and disbelief as I informed them I'd have to pass on their offer of a ticket to the athletics on the day of the 2012 London Olympics, that would come to be known as 'Super Saturday', because of the minor issue that my first working week would be capped off by a weekend of nights.

Aside from the staffing, starting on urology was also fortunate, because it meant my first on-calls would be in surgery. Understand this isn't because I was some budding knife-wielder – this was irrelevant, given the FY1 is unlikely to spend much time near theatre on call (or ever). As the dogsbody, and the person most recently having been at medical school (so likely to have forgotten the least of the non-cutty stuff), you're first port of call for handling most of the medical problems that arise on the wards out of hours. Which they do, since operations have a nasty tendency to trigger heart attacks and pneumonia in already delicate customers. Compared to medicine, there are a *hell* of a lot fewer surgical patients on the wards at any given time. For the same number of ward-cover doctors at night – a solitary FY1 – there were perhaps 70–100 inpatients, compared to up to 400 for the medical 'team' (the medical registrar and senior house officer were too busy in A&E to lend much of a hand).

Memories of the impossible task of medical ward cover still make me shudder. Medical ward cover FY1 in a hospital like this, for that many patients, is a job I'd have my work cut out to do well now, with years of experience. As a fledgling nudged out of medical school, it was often about survival – the junior doctor's, if not always the patients'.

The time before any night shift is accompanied by an inevitable nausea, gnawing in the stomach, as you're silently pulled towards the hospital with each hour and minute counted down.

Approaching the hospital, acceptance finally sets in, as the concrete obelisk of the main block erupts from the sprawl of dual carriageways and lost, patchy islands of green of suburbia's outskirts.

The shift would start with a handover meeting with the evening team – where the human fires already raging would be flagged. This would often be interrupted by multiple bleeps from anxious nurses, worried about their deteriorating patient, disbelieving when the response was simply: 'I'll add them to my list of several other possibly imminently dying patients and get to them as soon as I can.'

Not everything you get called about on a night shift is life or death, however – but you might not know that until you get there. I was once called to come urgently because a patient had something wrong with his eye. As hard as I tried, I couldn't get any more information than that and, assuming the worst, that he was at imminent risk of his eyeballs falling out and rolling across the ward, I headed over immediately. Arriving, I was greeted by a man in his sixties, sitting up in bed calmly. When I asked him what was wrong, he replied: 'It's this eye, doc, it feels funny.'

(Channelling Joe Pesci in *Goodfellas*:) 'Funny how? Can you see okay?'

'Yeah I can – the right one. Just sort of gritty.'

'Maybe like an eyelash?'

'Yeah, something like that.'

'Have you looked in the mirror?'

'Not yet . . .'

'Well how about we try that first, and if it's still a problem, we'll investigate further, maybe get the eye *surgeons* to have a look?'

I emphasised the word *surgeon* – with all of its connotations of scalpels becoming acquainted with eyeballs as strongly as I could – in the hope it might encourage him to sleep on it, rather than asking the nurse to call me back later. Before waiting for much more of a response, I turned and went to write in his notes.

'Patient reporting eye issue – ?eyelash.

Not for further investigation currently.

Plan: mirror.'

And then left before I could accidentally say something to the nurse, who had demanded I rush there, that would be against the 'treating colleagues with respect' policy.

Other times, the problem is just something no one knows quite what to do with. One night covering medicine, handover was cut short by the news that on the cardiology ward there was a patient whose implantable cardiac defibrillator (ICD) was misbehaving – in that it was overenthusiastically shocking him at random, sometimes several times per minute. To state what might seem obvious, this is not a nice experience. An ICD is a compact miniaturised version of the life-saving paddles beloved by shows like *ER*, implanted in a patient's chest, designed to kick in whenever the heart decides to go a bit jazz-fusion with the pumping rhythm – saving their life with the mysterious power of electricity. Great when it works, but each shock feels like getting punched squarely in the chest.

So there he was, lying in bed, but squared up to an invisible boxer, body blows landing unpredictably from the ether. To say he looked uncomfortable was an understatement. He stared up imploringly:

'You've got to do something about this . . .'

His sentence was interrupted by another phantom smack.

As soon as I've worked out what that something is, I'll get right on it, I thought but didn't say.

Fortunately (for me), the last discharge had left him semi-conscious, so he didn't notice my uncertain dithering. In this scenario, in theory you're simply supposed to deactivate the device by putting a magnet over it – stopping it from giving any more shocks. While this sounds simple, there is the underlying concern of 'what if the device isn't actually malfunctioning, but rather the patient's heart really is trying to kill them every 30 seconds and switching the ICD off finishes the job?' I'm sure any cardiologist reading this is tearing their hair out at this point, with a whole number of ECG and cardiac monitoring ways to tell the difference – but it's a little difficult to conjure these at the same time as focusing a chunk of your mental energy on not soiling yourself.

The other issue is getting your hands on the magnet. Apparently these should be readily available on the cardiology ward – but no one seemed to have one to hand.

Fortunately, before I had to contend any more with this, Simon the medical registrar turned up, having also heard about the patient in handover and (correctly) assuming this might be one that I was unable to handle solo.

'Have we got the magnet?' was Simon's immediate, breathless question.

'They're just looking for the keys to the cupboard.' The nurse in charge must have thought this would sound more reassuring than it did.

'Great, not like this is urgent or anything.'

We were interrupted inevitably by my bleep – meaning I'd have to leave Simon with the zap attack, saved by something much more comfortable and straightforward, like a patient deciding to bleed to death from their GI tract, a nice straightforward heart attack or similar.

* * *

In the notorious Essex town, when it came to letting off steam, newly ex-students barely had to break stride from their university days. The local leisure park was the imagined ideal – a concrete and glass monument to suburban diversion. Home to the essentials – a cinema, a Wild West decor-ed family restaurant and, most significantly, three nightclubs, each differently themed, yet somehow all the same. In what, as I repeat it now, sounds like a febrile, reckless combination of policies, the club offered free entry for NHS staff on Thursdays – and the drinks were three for the price of one all night. There was, of course, no option to buy a single drink. Shoes stuck and peeled off the dancefloor with each step, irony masking genuine enjoyment under the blanket of strobes and laser light beams.

The Thursday crowd was a strange mix of mainly hospital employees, combined with a diehard set of locals who couldn't wait for the weekend to get their fix. We treated one another with a wary curiosity. The divide would be bridged in the smoking area – a surprising number of doctors deciding they 'smoked when they drank', any health drawbacks offset by the opportunity to have a go at some 'community outreach', winning hearts and minds, and perhaps other areas. The response to these efforts would hover between 'you're actually alright' to 'my nan went into that hospital and never came out – they should just tear the whole fucking thing down'.

While I'd never suggest any of my colleagues were unprofessionally hungover at work the following day, I'm not sure Friday mornings were when the most dynamic work was done by many of them. One FY1 even allegedly 'procured' themselves a bag of IV fluids to re-hydrate overnight, only to hang it incorrectly and find in the morning it had fallen to the floor, with the effect that, thanks to gravity, he had inadvertently donated a pint of blood back into the bag.

Predictably, the place was also a sweaty incubator for ward romances. Most of these were short-lived, but there are also babies alive today who owe their very existence to the intoxicating blend of that drinks deal and 'Low' (or as everyone knows it, 'Apple Bottom Jeans') by Flo Rida.

The other face of this matchmaking coin could be seen on official hospital 'mess' nights – organised and subsidised by the social committee. What would begin with a relatively civilised meal would usually end up imaginatively at our regular haunt, or if we were feeling fancy, we'd venture further afield to the night club made famous by a reality show that will remain unnamed (but use your imagination). These nights would attract a wider cohort of the medical staff, including senior registrars with proper lives and even families, eager to run free in the nocturnal Essex wilderness. One orthopaedic specialist registrar (SpR) in particular could be seen gliding around the club, wedding ring oiled off his finger.

* * *

He was a cautionary example of the perils of extreme sports, in this case, impromptu Parkour (free running). The details were hazy, but apparently, while he and his friends were fleeing the police for unspecified reasons, he had confused video-game gravity with real life and thrown himself from an overpass, with leg-shattering consequences. Understandably, he wasn't keen to tell us any more about the accident than we already knew, perhaps because snitches get stitches, and he had already had enough of those. He had a nice new zipper running along the outside of his right thigh, where the orthopods (my new bosses, since rotating jobs) had gone in with their Meccano toy set, drilling a plate into his femur.

He was still under arrest, which in practical terms meant he was accompanied by two bored-looking police officers at all times. This was before smartphones were ubiquitous, so they spent most of their time re-reading that day's *Sun*, bickering with the patient and making cups of tea. For some of the time they had him in long looping escort restraints (less exciting than they may sound). This seemed excessive, given his leg, a likely key factor in a successful getaway, had just been operated on, and also his poor track record up to this point of actually escaping from the police.

The officers were very keen to know when he would be well

enough to leave hospital. That was a tough decision. On the one hand, he'd probably be fine if we – excuse my insensitive (given the location of his injury and his newfound mobility problem) choice of words – kicked him out there and then. On the other hand, jail isn't renowned for the intensive physiotherapy on offer after a broken leg, while also probably being a primo spot if you're in the market to pick up a post-operative infection. He was also pretty likeable – in many ways a bit naive, as we all can be at 19, but likeable, nonetheless. So we decided to keep him for a bit longer.

On first look, you might not have realised his dad's side of the family were Jamaican – I'd imagine he heard 'oh you look Mediterranean' more than once, minds cast back to their favourite holiday waiter, nationality unspecified. But growing up in this Essex slice of suburbia, I'm also pretty sure that, like Manchester United legend Ryan Giggs, he was black when it suited people. I say this as a person of mixed heritage, desperate for points of reference and role models to identify with growing up, who only found out Giggs's grandfather was Sierra Leonian after the story of Ryan sleeping with his brother's wife emerged. Suddenly every newspaper seemed to be running articles that highlighted his multicultural background.

'Safe for not sending me out.'

'It's fine – you do *probably* still need to be here . . . just about.'

The officers were outside the room at this point, so I could afford to be honest.

Satisfied I'd done my good deed for that hour at least, I headed to 'the office' – a small, windowless box with only two computers, shared with every other member of the happy multidisciplinary family on the ward. Hamish, the other FY1, was eating his lunch while hammering out discharge summaries for our more standard guests, octogenarians who had suffered collisions with the pavement – perfunctory sentences alternating with mouthfuls of whatever depressing filling he'd scraped between two slices of white bread (he was one of those 'food as fuel' psychos): 'Fell over, broke left hip, fixed with DHS (dynamic hip screw), had physio, went home' being the optimal length and level of detail if all went smoothly.

'I just saw Calvin.'

'Okay great, so we can take that off the list of jobs. Do you think he relates to you because you're . . .'

Hamish caught himself before finishing the sentence, but not before what he had meant to say had been made obvious.

'What, from Lewisham? Yeah it's basically like the film *Dangerous Minds* – I just go in there, turn my chair backwards and talk to him about the dangers of the street life.'

This didn't get much in the way of a response – possibly because *Dangerous Minds* is a reference that not even the film's theme song, perpetual banger 'Gangster's Paradise' can keep alive. Or, perhaps realising he was about to overstep the mark, he thought the better of continuing.

CHAPTER 2

Whiter than White Privilege

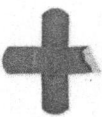

THE VOICE AT the end of the phone had notes of timid and apologetic, but a distinct lack of anything sounding like urgency.

'He's not moving or saying anything.'

'Well, it's night-time – are you sure he's not, you know . . . asleep?'

'I don't think so, but let me go and double-check.'

The phone went quiet for a few short but interminable moments, before a rustling heralded her return to the receiver.

'He's definitely not asleep.'

'Okay . . . is he alive? Is he for resus?'

The answer to this question is an important binary – whether a patient is felt to be fit enough for an attempt at resuscitation, or 'resus', decides whether they receive chest-shattering heroics or are allowed to pass away peacefully if their heart stops.

'I don't think so . . . no . . . not for resus. Please could you just come?'

By now it was clear that the time it would take to get a

clear story over the phone was at least double what it would take to walk there myself. And time wasn't currently a plentiful commodity. I had moved on to medicine, with the aforementioned quadrupling of the patient load during on-calls. After eight months on the wards, I at least knew the job a little, could actually be useful – but out of hours was still working well outside any sort of sane limit.

At night, when things are busy, dead patients present a conundrum when it comes to prioritisation. You definitely *do* have to go and see them – to confirm what everyone has already surmised, that the heart has stopped and the captain has abandoned the bridge. But how quickly? Certainly, some of the nurses would prefer you to come now, as would any neighbouring not-dead patients. The flimsy curtain around the bed does little to contain the gravitational waves of gloom radiating from the lifeless body.

On the other hand, the patient isn't getting any deader – and there is a list of others with body and soul still very much united to see. It's hard to put the dead ahead of the living, in case the delay helps nudge someone else over the line into the former category. Some nurses also have less of a problem hanging on to a less demanding patient for a while (they tend to leave the call bell alone). Once I come and confirm the death, the body is taken to the morgue, to be replaced by someone breathing with needs, pain, and functioning thumbs.

On this occasion, however, I didn't have anything that trumped the mortal riddle at the end of the phone. I headed along the exposed glass corridor that connected the main hulk of the hospital to the extra wards that had been bolted on, Frankenstein-style, as the local population aged and demand increased.

At night, lighting in the conduit was rationed using a motion sensor, illuminating only the occupied five-metre segment at any given time. In my delirium, there may have been times I convinced myself I was telekinetically responsible for the switch – accompanying each change with a flick of the wrist.

Arriving on the ward, the acute lack of frenetic activity answered the resus query pretty conclusively. The nurse in charge was sitting serenely in the glow of an anglepoise lamp, alternating between diligently scrawling in a breeze-block-sized set of patient notes and plucking Quality Street (fuel for a vast amount of NHS work among doctors and nurses alike) from a nearby tin.

'You called me about someone not responsive?'

'That was the other nurse, but yes, he's over there, bay one, bed three.'

She was a Nigerian woman in her early forties, part of the army of nurses originally from overseas that keep the hospital gears turning, especially overnight. Many have committed to the sort of working pattern that would make the most amphetamine-addled long-haul lorry driver weep – doing nights exclusively, to allow them to look after their kids in the daytime. Where sleep factors into this feat of endurance, I'm not sure.

In the bay, all of the beds were curtained off. An open ward can be as relaxing as a Download festival mosh pit. Understandably, many choose to drown out the sounds of wailing, snoring and thunderous commode use with whatever they can – music, a film, their own louder screams. Whether they use headphones for this often depends on a mix of their level of courtesy and the nurse in charge's efficiency as an enforcer. One neighbour was treating the ward to Magic FM classics, at what would under normal circumstances be considered obnoxious volume – but on this occasion was probably justified, given the person next to him had just died.

How much you talk to the dead in moments like these is something of a personal preference. I tend to check they're definitely not responding to their name, and leave it with that. As a registrar, I remember supervising one FY1, on the other hand, who talked the whole way through, explaining things in extra detail to the body, like he was soliciting for a particularly good YELP rating from beyond the grave. Each to their own.

'Mr Riley, can you hear me?'

I squeezed over his trapezius muscle to add a little emphasis. Nothing. So far, so dead. I looked under his lids, and the eyes already had the unmistakable clouded-glass quality that can be so shocking the first time you see it. The pupils, of course, remained slack and static when confronted by the light from my pen torch.

I put my stethoscope to my ears and pressed the bell to the waxy skin that stretched drum-like over the bone of his rib cage. No sound from within, I stood and everything was perfectly still for just a quiet moment. This soon passed, and my ears tuned back into the sound of the radio. Unmistakable twinkling droplets of guitar treble filled the air, soon joined by a voice so perfectly timed that I still struggle to believe it wasn't a fabrication of my addled brain.

'Hello darkness my old friend . . . I've come to talk with you again.'

* * *

During the days, on the care-of-the-elderly ward looking after medical patients not claimed by another specialty, the contrast in pace was palpable. There was still a mound of work to shift, but aside from the occasional emergency, it proceeded as a slow, methodical grind. The ward was all snow-capped scalps: we were caring for the most senior inpatients, admitted with infections or after falls (the final straw for their equilibrium) had toppled them and left them unable to cope at home.

These wards have an atmosphere that can at first be destab-ilising. It is often noisy – with the full-moon howls of those who have forgotten where they are and why, the wanderer stood by the door, patiently attended by a healthcare assistant, asking every new face who appears to let her out so they can 'just nip to the shops'. All of this is cut through sporadically by the smell – of laxatives or an enema finally working their intestinal magic.

Being the era of paper, we wheeled a cart of lilac folders across the squeaking, wipe-clean linoleum. The files were held in plastic hammocks suspended on hooked metal bars, with the major design flaw that these would twist, sometimes causing them to leave their runners, sending over-stuffed notes scattered in all directions. A significant chunk of the round would be spent delicately re-filing several decades' worth of medical history, inevitably shuffling the chronology.

Elderly care, geriatrics, medicine for older people – it is a speciality that has had to exist under many, ever-changing names. The constant rebranding is in significant part due to how society treats old people. Reference to advanced age runs the risk of offending – patients feeling it applies the label of frailty, decrepitude, senility. Perhaps we should try out 'antique'.

In reality, the spectrum of capability in the seventh decade and beyond is wide. Some are barely able to function, seeming as if the next breeze may be curtains for them, while there are others, however, who remain sharp, independent and dynamic – able to challenge the most overconfident of young upstart doctors on their reasoning. Where any of us will fall within this range is a function of genetics, class and how much fun we have eating, smoking and drinking earlier in life.

This state isn't static, even in the individual. The last five years have seen two men who would qualify for admission under geriatrics fiercely compete to be leader of the free world – only for time to catch up with Biden, leaving him shuffling and often seeming dazed and baffled, unsure where he is, let alone which country he's aiming the missiles at, eventually to be nudged aside by his own party. I say this as someone who almost certainly couldn't do any better in the job – but that's not the benchmark.

Now that they are skirting this age bracket, I am beyond grateful that my parents are in good shape, of sound mind – especially for the amount I'm still able to exploit them for free childcare and DIY assistance.

The demographic in this Essex hospital was, as you might imagine, very white and very working class. Every other man over the age of 60 was called Ron, which risked confusion (we almost had to number them, just to avoid making any lethal prescribing mistakes).

This is before considering the additional confounder of that generation's zany 'spin the wheel' approach to nicknames.

'Good morning, Mrs Elizabeth Cook?'

'I prefer Rose.'

'Oh, is that a middle name?'

This question is met with a blank face.

'No.'

She answers puzzled, like I'm the dickhead in this exchange. (And I can assure you, 'Peggy' is in no way short for 'Margaret', regardless of what anyone of that vintage may claim.)

It was the kind of environment where it wouldn't shock you if a patient referred to you as 'that nice coloured doctor' to their family – perhaps retro, certainly not ideal, but also without any air of real malice.

Whatever you call looking after the elderly, it is a speciality that falls under the category of 'thank God someone wants to do it'. It is the workhorse of inpatient general medicine, given that a large proportion of those sick enough to need to be in hospital are old.

I have heard the most glib and jaded doctors refer to care of patients with the most advanced dementia as 'veterinary medicine' – a sentiment that sounds unbelievably callous, grounds for GMC or even psychiatric referral. In many ways it is – but then again, we are a country that cares more about our pets than certain people, so perhaps the analogy could be worse.

The most charitable thing I can say about this comparison is that it's true that many patients can't tell you what is wrong – instead, it needs to be divined through intuition, and actually listening to the people who know them best. Much like in paediatrics, when their relatives or carers are worried, they're often right.

Another reason many of us are not enamoured with the realities of the speciality is that suddenly a whole host of things that seem to have very little to do with medicine become your problem.

Patient is a hoarder, and their house is a fire risk? Family want the whole place renovated, complete with walk-in jacuzzi and Louis XIV chandeliers, but don't want to pay for it? All of these and more will suddenly become obstacles preventing you from doing your job – which as an FY1 is getting people out the door, keeping the conveyor belt moving.

The geriatrics medical team sit in a carousel of meetings about their patients that go around and around, often with very limited opportunity for escape. The readiness for discharge bobs up and down – just as the nursing home place becomes available, some well-meaning idiot (me) decides to do a blood test, the result of which keeps them in, and the spot is gone. In more ways than one, residential and nursing homes can be like nightclubs (check the STI stats) – even if your name is down, you'll still have to wait a long time.

Some allied professions operate on completely different time-frames. In medicine, urgent means ideally now, or even better yesterday. In the world of social work it could mean days. Couple this with the fact that social workers are overburdened and understaffed, and the whole experience can feel like slow dental extraction.

If there are any young, idealistic medics reading this: please don't let me put you off – it's vital work, and I'm not itching to fill the gap. I'm assured by my career care-of-the-elderly colleagues there's a great deal they love about their jobs.

As much as we speak about underfunding of the NHS, its meagre, equally neglected twin is social care. I am in no doubt many of the admissions we have are caused by failures within this system – with inadequate visits contributing to immobility, missed meals and medication errors.

At the other end, patients are kept in waiting for care packages, or the aforementioned gold dust of a placement. Meanwhile, hospitals are dangerous places, filled with strange bacteria, no matter how much bleach we douse the place in. Hospital-acquired pneumonia may see them off long after they have been treated for whatever brought them in.

Anyone with elderly relatives, or a passing interest in the news, will be well aware of the fact that social care itself seems to be terminally ill. When told how much they'll need to contribute to costs, patients and families must think there is a decimal point in the wrong place.

A residential home placement in the UK costs on average between £800 and £1,070 per week, while nursing homes are around £1,200–1,400. That is more than the entire take-home salary of a full-time NHS consultant.

If you have no savings and don't own your own home,

then costs are paid for. Anything above £23,000 stashed away (including the value of your home if moving into a facility), however, and you'll foot the bill. Many people are forced to sell their homes, and everything built up over a lifetime working is quickly vapourised.

I don't want to dent my progressive credentials too much by dying on the hill of rights for inheritors – if the rest of society worked the way it should, none of this would be a problem. But we now have a situation where it has become the only realistic means of passing on some kind of security. People should no doubt contribute, but the idea of penalising the sick in this way also feels unfair.

Care in your own home isn't much better – although at least your house isn't at risk, just any savings. A bigger problem, however, is having no one to actually deliver whatever care package the occupational therapist might think a patient needs. Thanks to low wages and visa restrictions, there isn't quite the queue of people from abroad lining up to do the washing, dressing and wiping we have all become accustomed to outsourcing.

There are currently tens of thousands of vacancies in the care sector, with often little appetite among the British-born to clean British backsides. In the past, we would have filled these spaces with workers from overseas, but now earnings thresholds have been increased, and migrants are prohibited from bringing dependents. This is amid the current fixation and rhetoric around migration, the net effect being we are losing out on an essential part of the workforce.

Given the costs above, some families opt to keep their relatives out of care for as long as possible – taking on the tasks themselves. If they can manage it, the savings would arguably make them among the highest-paid care workers in the world.

Some communities are more set up for this than others. The intergenerational households more common among South Asian families, for example, anecdotally at least, seem to push back the point at which living at home is no longer viable.

* * *

When treating patients in the later stages of dementia, it can feel almost impossible to do what is right. Without wanting to sound callous, so much of the person that was once there is often gone, or is at least trapped, wandering and lost, smothered by a blanket of inner fog. The repertoire of speech withers, until a couple of phrases or words are all that is left, sometimes even just a sound, stripped of all language. These still penetrate deeply and leave their mark. I can recall the exact tone of one woman's voice, whose only refrain towards the end was the endless repetition of 'please no more!' – regardless of what was being done for her.

We were approaching the door of the room of one similarly incapacitated patient. The geriatrics ward round that Thursday morning consisted solely of me and Mike, the consultant. Unusually for the time (a lot has changed, even in 12 years), he was a boss who insisted on first-name terms with his juniors. This practice prompted a raised eyebrow from the more hierarchical orthopaedics consultants on my previous rotation – they often solicited Mike's help to ensure they didn't break too many fragile grandparents in the pursuit of joint and femur fixing.

Whenever he wanted an opinion on medical care for his patients, Mr Foster, the king of hips, would ask: 'Why don't you go and ask *Mike* . . .'

The word 'Mike' was inflected with just the correct amount of derision to make clear to me that if I ever made the mistake of thinking *we* were on first-name terms, *my* bones would be the ones needing resetting.

As consultants go, Mike was young, idealistic and eccentric – gliding around the wards in a three-piece suit, complete with pocket watch. Coupled with a side parting, he looked like a widow's locket photo of her sweetheart, lost at the Somme. Looking out of time, he was also out of place – he had a background in academic medicine (having completed a PhD during training), but had forgone the bastions of science and specialism in favour of making a difference at the great grey coal face. But this was a case that had been stretching even him to the limit. We braced ourselves, and entered the room.

Inside, there was the staleness that is common to hospitals and the bedrooms of teenagers – even with diligent cleaning, it is hard to be fully rid of it when a sweating body festers in the bed for much of the day. The blinds were closed, the dim light enhancing the sense that we were crossing into a lair.

'Nggghhh . . .'

As she groaned, she would intermittently sit up, jerking like an animatronic theme park attraction. A tiny, frail woman of 78 years, wild smoke-white hair exploded from her skull as her eyes raked the room, never truly fixing on anything.

She was completely non-verbal – although her family assured us she was normally much better. I was inclined to believe them, because looking after her in her current state was more than the nurse and 1:1 healthcare assistant could cope with, so God knows how they would have managed at home. Her loved ones had done one of the best things possible – filled the room with pictures of the person she was, her and her many children and grandchildren, smiling, wearing her own clothes. Although it shouldn't be necessary, the humanity gazing out from the photos kept watch against moments where it might otherwise be forgotten.

Despite being able to do absolutely nothing for herself, some fragment of consciousness, coupled with sheer determination, allowed her to locate and quickly rip out any IV cannula soon after it was put in – the FY1's proudest, most fraught work dashed in an instant. The fact that she was also not drinking meant she was becoming what one of the more irreverent geriatricians referred to as 'crispy dry' – the surface of her lips looked like Alpen.

Patients stopping eating and drinking is a normal part of dying – the processes are ultimately mutually exclusive. This may seem obvious, but convincing a family that a loved one's life is coming to an end, on the other hand, can be much more challenging.

In the room was one of her daughters – a polite but direct woman in her mid-forties, the corners of her eyes prematurely wrinkled by cigarette smoke, accompanied by her son. He was more animated; in his twenties, he sprang from his chair in the corner when we entered and paced around while we spoke.

As we conveyed our belief that Josephine was coming to the end of her life, and that we didn't feel there was much that more intervention would achieve, the conversation had quickly become intense.

'Doctor, if she just had something to eat, surely she'll get her strength back – and she might get better . . . Couldn't you put a tube down?'

It's hard to argue with this sort of logic, but there's little evidence that being more invasive would improve things, and the cycle of her yanking it out of her nose, only for us to have to wrestle and stuff it back in, wouldn't be good for anyone's health – hers, or ours.

'It doesn't really work like that . . .'

'But she's strong, she's a fighter. You *have* to do everything you can.'

Wheeling out statistics and studies and pitting them against the emotion of Granny dying, you've already lost. This can be the case with any family – but when the granny in question is the cast-iron matriarch of an Irish traveller family, one that has kept four generations in check, it's next to impossible.

Medically, there wasn't much hope – we had treated the urine infection that had been our best guess, hedging our bets and using antibiotics that covered pretty much everything else as well.

'You can't just give up on her.'

This wasn't said with menace – but it did convey the truth, that if we weren't careful, didn't provide the best, we would regret it. In situations like these, the spectre of the PALS (Patient Advice and Liaison Service) office looms, ostensibly there to mediate between medical teams and families – but often in reality serving as the gateway to a complaint.

* * *

Given the understandable mistrust of institutions by many traveller families, a lot of what doctors say may sound like simply not caring. And there can often be friction, which can lead to genuine discrimination. As in many communities, when things aren't looking good, extended families can arrive to keep a vigil, with any disagreements over care or access raising the possibility of conflict with staff.

The treatment of travellers in wider society tests the concept of white privilege to the limit. At best, they may be granted some grace from a distance, but I can think of no other group that seems to forfeit it so quickly once they open their mouths. Many establishments may as well have left up their 'no Irish' signs, and just clarified exactly who they mean with an asterisk.

Spend time in suburbia or the country long enough, and you

will hear people talking about travellers in polite company in terms that, if used about other groups, would prompt terminal public shaming. In my secondary school, the other 'P word' was bandied around as an insult for anyone – it could land on you for almost anything, from having holes in your shoes to stealing a car.

This idea that criminality permeates all corners of the traveller community is so set in the minds of some that it is resistant to almost all reason and, of course, statistics to the contrary. Present the idea that crime is likely driven by deprivation and lack of opportunity, and to match rates in other comparable communities, you'll be labelled naive and terminally liberal.

Something the travelling community have working against them is visibility, particularly among those who still move regularly. Every group, regardless of ethnicity or economic status, contains a minority of arseholes, but they will draw attention whenever they arrive in new places. Prejudice against travellers also ignores the fact that the vast majority of those identifying as travellers now live in a single location, with the vast majority remaining out of sight of the curtain twitchers with such strong opinions.

Health outcomes among travellers are shocking. The baseline life expectancy is 10–12 years lower than the national average. One estimate from 2007 (and admittedly outside the UK) determined that, in the Dublin area, 50 per cent of travellers died before their 40th birthday. Those are developing world numbers, among people supposedly with access to the same resources as everyone else.

A few things seem to drive these headlines. Death in childhood is much more common – some sources suggest as many as 10 per cent of traveller children die before their second birthday.

Accidents, especially on roads, disproportionately affect travellers – particularly men, which, combined with a high suicide rate, puts a massive dent in their longevity statistics.

An obvious measure of how excluded any group is, is to ask when was the last time you saw one of their members in a position of power. Currently, could you imagine the prime minister being a traveller? Less ambitiously, when was the last time you met a doctor, lawyer, or any other of the go-to professions who identified as a member of the traveller community? You haven't, because they're barely out there. Sindy Joyce, the first traveller to receive a PhD from an Irish university, was headline news in 2019.

At the risk of sounding like a warped and skipping 45 record, this is not the result of some intrinsic flaw or deficiency. It is the inevitable outcome when a group are excluded from wider society – even while allowing for and acknowledging historic lifestyle differences that may contribute to the distance from the mainstream.

I say all of this clearly, not as a member of this community, but as part of a healthcare system that owes travellers better. Anything I'm writing needs to be accompanied by (and indeed superseded by) the voices of travellers themselves.

Nothing I have said should be taken as questioning the validity of the concept of white privilege in wider contexts. This is not some desperate play for conservative acceptance, blinkered by individual prosperity. Anyone who holds up a particular group of disadvantaged white people as evidence that it doesn't exist is either being disingenuous or thick. It should be clear that the simple fact of being non-white can hold people back in many situations, while not negating the many other forms of oppression – and there are very few situations, if any, where it doesn't impact experience in some way, however small.

I will leave the naysayers to google 'intersectionality'. Suffice to say that while being a traveller is no doubt difficult in myriad ways, if, however, thanks to the gift of multiculturalism, a traveller also happens to be black, life might end up being a whole lot more challenging.

* * *

In situations like the one facing us with Josephine, being dogmatic is rarely the answer. Times, and therefore medical evidence and trends, change, leaving your rigid faith looking absurd in hindsight. You don't want to be the guy who died on the 'Betamax is best' hill. When it leads you to butt against a patient and their family for no clear gain, it can also be damaging in the here and now.

At the time, there was a trend from some consultants towards militantly resisting any requests from families for IV hydration once their relatives had stopped drinking. In this case, a drip clearly wasn't the answer, but rather than a flat no, Mike suggested we would be happy to try one more IV, but asked the family to stay and help keep her calm.

Witnessing her distress at even just the attempt at another cannula was enough for the family to accept we shouldn't put in any more, once this one inevitably fell out. There was no fight, no threats of lawyers, just a skilful manoeuvre to get everyone on the same page.

The ward round moved on – we had another bay to trudge through, before the discharge meeting beckoned. I was spared by the bleep. When I returned from the phone, I mustered an exaggerated hangdog expression. Maria, the registrar, had finished going round the other half of the patients.

'Sorry, it's the third time downstairs have called – I need to get down there before they close at five, or I'll be on the slab next to Mrs Rivers.'

Maria scowled, but knew she couldn't do anything about it – my absence meant she would be forced to scribe in the meeting, documenting the plans which would inevitably collapse and come to nothing.

Geriatric medicine is where young doctors become most familiar, most comfortable with death and dying. This is reflected in a little-publicised quirk of hospital work – cremation forms. For reasons including the disturbing fact that there is a risk of explosion if patients are cremated with pacemakers still in place, showering the congregation with gruesome, unwanted mementos, a doctor needs to check and sign off that it is safe to incinerate a body.

I still don't fully understand why, but at the time, this was considered extra work outside of normal responsibilities. Doctors were paid a small additional fee for doing the form (don't worry, nowhere near enough that some psychopath was going to start testing the limits of the Hippocratic oath for financial gain). The windfall had picked up the distasteful nickname 'Ash Cash' – and, on this occasion, I was essentially being paid extra not to sit through the meeting.

By virtue of the cohort of patients admitted to our ward, and their proclivity for dying (expectedly, not because I was especially useless), I became familiar with the staff in the euphemistically titled 'Patient Affairs' office. The place where death's admin is done. They had their work down to a well-oiled process – greasing the wheels with cups of tea and polite persistence. This was required, as, similarly to the on-call conundrum, during the day, the living also demand attention, relegating the dead to the bottom of the priority list. Doctors could be slow to come, and families understandably get even more upset if the hospital hoards their relatives after failing to keep them alive.

Sue and Elaine had the sort of unnerving cheeriness that can feel out of place, but isn't uncommon among those working in the business of death. They were well suited to dealing with errant medics, and had taken steps to pre-empt our blunders. A laminated example copy of a correctly filled-out form was stuck to the wall – presumably after one too many bodies had been held up due to our inability to tick the correct box about the person in the box.

Alongside the cremation form, there is the death certificate. If anything, this exerts more gravity, feels more weighty. It is the record preserved forever, or at least until society crumbles, of the final punctuation to a life. Sometimes it's obvious what killed someone – they were doing a Sudoku, had a massive aneurysm, dead.

With older people, often with multiple vying long-term illnesses, it can be closer to a *Murder on the Orient Express* scenario. All of them have stuck in the blade, and choosing a prime suspect feels arbitrary. Do we blame the urinary tract infection, that then caused sepsis? Or the heart attack they had a week into treatment?

Once completed, we would present our work to them for inspection, waiting breathlessly – like a child with a spelling test.

'You can't have "Old Age" as a cause of death.'

'But why not? It would make everything *so* much simpler – I could just get a stamp – they're all *really* old.'

Even though everything could have accurately been classified as a disease of ageing, they are of course correct. Normally the cause is decided by the consultant, but ultimately, we learned to keep it simple. Did they have the illness, and is it a plausible thing that might have killed them? Good enough.

* * *

Back at the house, in the early July sun, Dave was wallowing in the ridiculous oversized paddling pool he had bought, clutching a Corona. The grass around him remained long and overgrown thanks to a wet spring, combined with our laissez faire attitude to mowing (we were early rewilders, against the wishes of the landlady).

The feeling of that first year of work now feels alien – where, regardless of how intense the hours in the hospital were, time away from work was truly free. We were simultaneously buoyed by a new elevated professional status (above being medical students at least), without the pressure yet of having to truly make something of ourselves. Hours in the evening were in need of filling, rather than squeezed as they are now, wrung out for every last drop of productivity between childcare and work.

The host of still juvenile medics that descended on these Essex suburbs may have supposedly been upstanding members of society, but this didn't mean we moved in without leaving a mark. When it came time for us to leave, Dave's poor man's hot tub left a perfect circle of swampy ground, and the garden was a mess.

Although it was hardly a ruin, the landlady was less than pleased, and when it came time to leave at the end of the year, the predictable tug of war over the deposit followed. Maybe they should add 'no junior doctors' to that sign.

* * *

The on-call rota, peppered with blocks of weekends, nights and sporadic evenings of ward cover here and there, means there is rarely a week without some such obligation. Taking a holiday is close to impossible without an often-complex series of swaps – making the summer pass by like any other season, enhancing that universal sensation of never grasping it fully, lost through your fingers.

The knowledge that we would be rotating to new hospitals the first week of August brought forward and amplified that 'back to school' atmosphere, the subtle grief that descends in late summer, a time when every warm evening feels like the last night of the fair.

Best not tug too hard on the thread as to why I was slumming it at a house party thrown by my brother, a fifth-year medical student – but I was there, taking in the hedonism by osmosis, unconstrained as they were by the realities, anxiety and slog of their final year for another month, before the cold splash of September's new term hit them.

The flat was in an ex-council block in Shoreditch, the rooms considered suitably dingy that the producers of the TV show *Luther* had once used their place as a location – the lair of a particularly insalubrious wrong 'un.

It was an every-room-packed, beats-blasting-from-battling-aux-cable-DJs, bodies-spilling-out-onto-the-walkways affair. If I lived next door now, it would have me glaring out of the window in a dressing gown.

Given my hapless track record, it was a blessing that Louise approached me, rather than vice versa – removing the need for anything that might resemble suave on my part. Suffice to say, without being overly modest, beautiful women sauntering across the room unprompted and making it clear they were interested in me wasn't a daily occurrence.

Before you trouble yourself too much with the mental arithmetic of appropriateness (or the creep's calculus if you prefer), I'll point out for my reputation's sake that Louise was a graduate student – and we were exactly the same age.

We spent the rest of the night at the party together – mercifully this was a PG-rated affair, given she's also a doctor, and no doubt one day our children will read this (although perhaps I'm deluded in my belief they'll be interested). It ended with us going for a walk and lying under a tree on the scrap of grass in front of the tower, a romantic stroll through a housing estate.

Our first real date a couple of weeks later came a few days after my triumphant return to London, belongings packed into the aforementioned leaking Corsa. She has since admitted that thanks to my lackadaisical text etiquette, she wasn't even sure I would show up. Apparently, my immature communication skills had me unintentionally playing hard to get – something that couldn't have been further from the truth.

I opted for a painfully cool cocktail bar and instantly paid the price. Above the steps down to the basement was an infamous Glenn Ligon canvas, *No Room* – against a gold background, in black type, quoting Richard Pryor, it reads:

'I was a nigger for twenty-three years.

I gave that shit up. No room for

No room for advancement'

Whatever you may think of the piece, the effect was jarring out of context, or rather displayed in this new one – a place owned by a white celebrity chef, apparently keen to show he was 'down', much like the white guy rapping along to the parts of a Wu Tang song he shouldn't.

You're left imagining the various responses of all those around, deprived of the little white card at the museum to give a helping hand in understanding, and so left to come to their own conclusions (like, 'hey maybe this is funny, perhaps I can even *say* it!'). Or perhaps they catch the eye of one of the few black people present, eyebrow raised, seeking some opinion or approval.

Once downstairs, drinking cocktails that neither of us could afford, but I would be paying for (she was still a student after all), we played a game of musical chairs as the staff seated and then re-seated customers repeatedly, in an effort to squeeze groups into the oversubscribed space.

But none of this mattered. It was the sort of evening where I can in no way remember to tell you exactly what we talked about – only there were no unintended silences.

CHAPTER 3

Back Once Again

AFTER THE COMFORT of being unambiguously bottom of the pile as an FY1, the promotion that follows, to FY2, is a no man's land. In old money, I was now a senior house officer, or 'SHO' – a doctor who has safely (or safely enough) navigated their first year without proving too lethal, and so is now worthy of full registration with the GMC.

In reality, this just means being shunted to the bottom of a new pile – the SHO phase runs for at least three years (the later two coming after being accepted onto a specialty training programme), until the dizzy heights of registrar are reached. So, in continuing on their rotations, FY2s find themselves on the same rota, doing the same work as and being compared to doctors with more experience – and who have actually chosen to train and work in the given specialty.

Safely back in London, I was at a hospital we'll call the Citadel – an imposing fortress of a building, a hybrid of architectural eras, with modern utilities roughly grafted onto a fading regency trunk. It was the kind of well-resourced centre of excellence where pampered professors carve out fiefdoms, while looking down their noses at their poor provincial counterparts.

In a place filled with egos, where prima donnas expect things to be done to the highest of standards (their way or not at all), the odd tantrum is inevitable. The management had thought of an ingenious way of appearing to address this, without actually doing anything about it.

'And remember, we absolutely do *not* tolerate bullying.'

During this five-minute induction video, they had spoken about bullying more than an episode of *Sesame Street* aimed at teaching kids to play nicely. This level of focus on the issue wasn't reassuring – like the restaurant a little too keen to tell you about their hygiene standards: 'Our chefs *always* wash their hands . . . no food poisoning here!'

In any case, I would be starting on cardiology – lucky for me it's not a specialty with a reputation for type-A narcissists, public humiliation and psychopathy . . . (for balance, there are plenty of perfectly civil cardiologists out there).

Creature of habit as I am, the hospital also happened to be one of the main teaching sites for the medical school from which I had graduated the previous year – and which both Louise and my brother still attended. It would be entirely possible that either of them could be attached to the ward I was working on, opening up a host of professionalism and HR dilemmas, imagined or real. Then again, medicine is a small world, and this situation was hardly unique – it wouldn't be unheard of to find domestic tensions aired in theatre between romantically entwined surgeon and anaesthetist, played out one passive-aggressive request to 'raise the bed slightly' at a time.

I may have taken the need to retain an air of professionalism a little too far, however. If she senses herself losing an argument, Louise will still bring up the time during this rotation when I (perhaps overzealously) shooed her away from the ward when she came up to say hi. I was apparently worried that social visits were the first step on a treacherous slope ending in malpractice and prison. She had messaged to see what I was up to – predictably this was sitting in the office with the two FY1s, alternating between writing discharge summaries and bothering other specialties to come and review our patients (usually the diabetes team, given the tendency of over-sweetened blood to crystallise in coronary arteries).

'What are you up to?'

I stepped out of the door of the ward, rather than inviting her in.

'I'm busy . . .'

'Saving lives? Looks like an episode of *ER* in there.'

She gestured inside to the empty corridor, in visual terms a veritable hive of inactivity – although possibly an unfair characterisation, since even in cardiology, at the junior levels, most of the work *is* admin.

'You could just say you're teaching me, taking me – a *medical* student – to see patients at this *teaching* hospital.'

'People might still talk.'

'And say what? That you're doing your job?!'

'That it's inappropriate!'

'Fine, I'll go.'

This was delivered in a tone that indicated unequivocally that it *wasn't* fine, and that we would be discussing this again later – but I let her go anyway. This sort of paranoia about imagined, unpredictable consequences from the bosses was the net result of a culture where you could be hauled up at any point, for seemingly innocent things.

Louise had recently moved into a flat owned by a classmate five minutes from the hospital – one that was nicer than anything I could hope to afford, even as a consultant, let alone an SHO. The perks of hanging out with people from 'comfortable' families. The ample light flooding through bay windows, high ceilings and period features, coupled with the convenience, meant I spent almost as much time there as I did in my flat – the aforementioned shooing incident having not been quite enough to consign me to the relationship landfill. Comparatively, my place (in her opinion, not mine) was a hovel in the depths of Dalston.

This rehearsal of domesticity was interrupted when, as is the case for all final-year students, she was shipped off to one of the linked district general hospitals. These stints serve as a prelude to the upheaval of the foundation experience, with the added discomfort of hospital accommodation, which is everything you'd imagine it to be. These places tend to resemble the most neglected student halls of residence, all visible breeze blocks and MDF furniture.

During this period, deprived of the option of a quick stroll to hers (I truly am a martyr), my commute was a multi-train trip home from the hospital's genteel postcode back into the depths of east London, infuriatingly passing many closer hospitals on the way. Somehow I could never manage to align living and working within the same compass segment.

I ended with a walk along Dalston high street, the archetype for the changes in London – gentrification a tide that laps against the bedrock, but also erodes. Natural wine bars wedged in between pound shops and phone repair kiosks, old Rastas riding bikes along the pavement, blue plastic bag of yams dangling from the handlebars.

Turning on to Ridley Road, you could be in another country –

not in the huffing, 'I don't recognise Britian anymore' sense, but rather stepping into a place where the dial has been moved up a notch on all of your senses. More accurately, you're in many countries all at once.

There are West African aunties wheeling caddies laden with the day's shopping – plantains bartered down in a game of wills with the stall owner. They might stop at a table selling head wraps, every imaginable colour laid out, a menagerie adorning incongruously pale-hued, disembodied mannequin heads. This all side by side with the old East Enders, selling suspiciously cheap bowls of fruit, melons 'two for a pound'.

It's a part of London that has at times attracted lurid coverage. A quick search will find you articles about a minority of butchers on the road, who catered to tastes for meats not deemed up to food safety standards, selling 'smokies' and bush meat under the table. It is also the setting and filming location for the show *Top Boy*, and while gangs, drugs and the associated violence undoubtedly have a presence, this extreme depiction unfairly tarnishes the area.

In our nearby flat, the dank semi-basement and first floor of what must once have been a beautiful townhouse, we were part of the problem: moving in, paying above the odds so we could be near a place where things were 'happening' at the weekend, in a vain attempt to cling to our youths – and in the process contributing to driving out locals who had given the place its soul.

* * *

The jolt momentarily stiffened all of his muscles, audibly moving the bed, the rigour followed by a zombie-like rousing. As he flexed forward, his arms flailed and his eyes rolled back, the restored rhythm of his heart not yet having returned enough blood to his brain to bring it back online fully. Instead, he was running on the base-level programming – simple functions such as breathing, moaning and lashing out at perceived threats (nursing staff) were intact, but not a great deal else.

Ideally when shocking someone during an arrest, they've already been tubed and put to sleep, protecting us from this sort of pummelling – but not on this occasion. His heart had stopped while attached to a monitor, surrounded by doctors and nurses, minutes after being wheeled up from his angiogram – meaning he was brought back within seconds, use of his limbs intact. A real hospital pass from the interventional team downstairs.

As other members of the team variously attempted to calm, restrain and push drugs into him, I stood hovering by the defibrillator. I waited for the neat, ordered trace on the monitor 'compatible with life' to degenerate into the erratic, childlike scrawl of fibrillation, as it had several times already – to the point that the novelty of resurrecting him Lazarus-like had almost worn off, replaced by a sense of tedious repetition. It's important not to let the mind wander and miss the next rhythm that needs shocking. No one wants to be responsible for a man's death because they were too busy debating whether to have pizza, Thai or Indian for that Friday evening's takeaway.

As suddenly as he had popped up, he slumped back down to the bed.

Slightly wearily, Benas, the SpR, called out, 'Okay, he's gone again, rhythm check.' (This refers to assessing the regularity (or otherwise) of the heartbeat, rather than a measure of how badly you'll embarrass your kids when you hit the dancefloor at a wedding.)

'It's VF[1] again, everyone else clear, oxygen away.' This well-

---

1   Jittery disordered electrical activity in the heart – ominously termed incompatible with life – an indication for a life saving shock.

rehearsed sequence of instructions is designed to minimise the risk of killing a colleague, either by shocking them directly, or creating a fireball – never a good career move, and there's a lot of paperwork involved.

This level of excitement in the body, and therefore the patient's room, following a heart attack isn't uncommon. The bruised and potentially scarred cardiac muscle interferes with the normal electrical transmission, allowing upstart fibres away from the normal pacemaker to start firing off nonsensical rhythms, like a drunk commandeering the conductor's podium at the Philharmonic.

This situation could in theory have gone on indefinitely. When someone's heart has stopped completely, after a prolonged period of trying and failing to restart, the furtive glances start and eventually things are called off, as all agree it's looking futile. Not that you'd want to, but it's poor form to do this when the miracle drug that is direct current is still proving effective in bringing the patient back, even if just momentarily.

It's bizarre we don't comment more on how useful electricity is as a treatment for our most vital of organs: heart stops working, we just plug you into the mains, flip the switch and hope for the best (for legal reasons I am obliged to say it's a little more complicated than that, and please don't try this with the sockets at home).

On this occasion, the drugs seemed to finally do their thing – probably the amiodarone that was now hanging from the drip stand (a note to medical students facing a grilling: in the short term, because it treats a wide array of rhythms, amiodarone is rarely a *completely* wrong answer – although long term, less ideal, as it has as many side effects as the number of conditions it treats). My hovering, Zeus-like finger didn't need to dispense another thunderbolt, and after a few minutes, the apparatus of the resuscitation team was disassembled.

A while later, the cardiology consultant arrived back on the ward to inspect the battlefield and engage in some morale-boosting shouting. He was a short, intense, bald man, whose mood could be gauged by the grinding of his teeth. Now, his jaw was in overdrive, a violent churn of clenching and unclenching, the movement accentuating the vessels that bulged at his temples. His tanned skull glistened like an angry conker. Cardiology can be the most false-macho among the otherwise often bookish physician-ly specialties – all intervention, steely glares and crotch-thrusting bravado.

The registrar, Benas, was a locum over from Lithuania doing a short run of shifts, despite already being a consultant back home. The escalated pay and apparently favourable pre-Euro exchange rate at the time meant it was still worth the sacrifice of leaving his family, suffering the ignominy of demotion and the tempest of emotions that was a Dr Scott ward round.

Benas was straightforward, almost to the point of being unreadable. He seemed to do almost nothing while over in the UK, other than come in to work, before heading home to his Travelodge, via Tesco, where he stocked up on the cold sandwiches that apparently made up his every depressing meal. He had the spartan, routine existence of some mild-mannered serial killer.

'How's the chap from earlier?'

The concern and bonhomie that might have been conveyed by Dr Scott's question was undermined by his tone and the past two months of excoriation. It was understood that any answer less than 'fine – almost well enough to dance off the ward' would be met with fury. We couldn't allow the inconvenience of post-procedure complications to jeopardise the shiny new stent he had just artfully placed in this man's vessel. Fortunately, the patient's heart was now behaving – producing nice tedious predictable traces on the monitor, and he was sleeping (the nurses assured us of this, regardless of *how* dead he may have looked).

'He's much better – he was just awake and chatting to his wife.'

'Excellent, perhaps we're not all completely useless then.' This is what passed for a pat on the head.

First bullet dodged, but with plenty still left in the clip, attention turned to the rest of the ward. Another patient who had also had a heart attack was in the coronary care unit (CCU) and his had been sufficiently large, that this heart muscle was no longer able to pull (or push) its weight. Interventional cardiologists like toys – and some may bring them in to play even when the evidence for benefit is borderline. This man had a balloon on the end of a catheter sitting in his aorta, inflating and deflating in time with his heart. This apparently helps with pumping and blood supply, although without a great deal of proof that it actually stops patients from dying after an MI (of course I say this as a non-cardiologist, so what do I know?).

Having a balloon floating around in the main conduit between your heart and the rest of your body longer than is necessary isn't a good idea. The plan had been, that assuming our man had the decency to remain stable, the pump would be removed by this afternoon. Best-laid plans being what they are, thanks to our earlier heroically time-consuming efforts to keep the other customer alive, it remained, bobbing around in his aorta.

The anger that greeted this update almost seemed to be burnished with glee – at having caught us out and permitting him to exorcise his pent-up rage.

'So the pump is still there? Even though I *clearly* said this morning it was to come out!?'

As can be the case with high-stress, high-prestige jobs that attract type-A, academically gifted individuals, medicine has the tendency to create tyrants. Without the risk of physical retribution that unquestionably accompanied their school years, these alpha-nerds have free rein to berate their underlings. So, this is how the 6ft 2 Benas found himself looming over the Napoleonic figure of Dr Scott, and having to put up with the unjustified hairdryer treatment without slapping him. His only choice was to take it, and calmly, almost robotically, state the facts.

'The pump is still in because we were dealing with the other patient.'

Although true, this didn't seem to be a satisfactory answer.

'You mean you can't look after more than one fucking patient at a time? There's a whole ward here.'

'No, but this man was very sick . . .'

Dr Scott glared, unmoved by this perfectly logical explanation.

'We're in a hospital . . . Everyone here is very sick. Well, don't just stand around here – go and take it out.'

Benas broke his stare – any upset at being chastened and spoken to like a child for things beyond his control offset by the permission to disappear. He headed to the storeroom to get the necessary equipment to take out the balloon, while presumably fantasising about ways of using the guidewire and scalpel to make Dr Scott's heart stop.

* * *

Staring out from the wall, he had his serious face on – Captain America jawline resolutely fixed and confronting the scourge of healthcare tourism. 'NHS hospital treatment is not free for everyone' read the stern inscription. This poster, and others like it, hangs in almost every hospital I have worked in. They foreshadow the visit from the 'Overseas Team' who scour the hospital for non-UK residents, and once a potential chargeable patient is deemed well enough, will descend to see what they can squeeze out of their pockets.

The cost of health tourism to the UK goes up and down in prominence, depending on how badly the NHS is doing, and where we are in an election or referendum cycle. Back in the heady days of Brexit campaigning, one side painted visitors as the stowaways weighing us down, while the other suggested their rivals were making feathers out to be lead, and that the small amount that could be clawed back was negligible.

Predictably, I think the truth most likely lies somewhere in the middle. The cost of treating migrants (regardless of status) to the UK is real. It's probably also not massive, and is difficult to offset accurately against other factors including taxes paid by legal visitors.

A figure of £1.4 billion per year is given as the cost of migrants using NHS services, but the majority of this is visitors who pay tax, and are visiting from countries with reciprocal health-care agreements with the UK. There is the immigrant health surcharge – a specific additional payment designed to cover these costs. At the last reliable (pre-Brexit) estimate, actual health tourism, with money and resources draining away, likely accounted for 0.3 per cent of the NHS budget.

Recently, outside of the *Daily Mail*, it doesn't seem to have been such a hot topic, perhaps because the NHS is now in such a state that fewer people would bother coming here in the hope of 'stealing healthcare' – like breaking into a car with no steering wheel and a family of squirrels living under the bonnet.

If anything, more British patients are having to resort to going abroad themselves, to places such as Turkey, for sun, sea and surgery, rather than languish on waiting lists for over a year.

Fortunately, it's not my job to identify these patients, but they can be forgiven for being suspicious. When a patient's awake, it's much easier to find out a little more about them, and I took the opportunity to take a proper history from Mr Maseko, the unfortunate man to whom I had been giving the electrode treatment earlier.

'Where were you born?'

At this, his brow furrowed.

'Why do you want to know that?'

This question had clearly soured things and I quickly scrabbled to justify myself.

'Sorry . . . it's just certain things you're exposed to growing up can affect the diseases you get now.'

He looked sceptical, but I hoped I had at least part-way convinced him I was asking him this for his own good, rather than out of some vigilante border guard compulsion.

He was originally from Malawi – my infectious disease colleagues would no doubt have instantly become tumescent at that titbit, although they would presumably have already been able to divine not only the country, but the specific village, just from the patient's name. And, of course, yes, he swam in the lake as a child. Schistosomiasis parasites picked up from the water can find their way into the lungs, and from there back up blood flow to the heart, eventually causing heart failure.

Now, was this the cause of his current predicament? Almost certainly not. Overeager medical students and new doctors learn quickly that it's almost always the mundane answer: in this case, 40 years of exposure to the glorious excesses of a Western diet and smoking, coupled with genetics, had landed him here. But it is still relevant, and questions that might affect the quality of a patient's care can easily become loaded.

It would be convenient to go on to tell you that, at this point, he opened up. Although he had been in the UK for much of his adult life, he came alive when discussing his first home. Walking to the village school with his friends, running away from the elders when they had been up to no good, his mother's cooking, church on Sunday. Unfortunately (for me) this tangent to our conversation never happened; there was no life-affirming reminiscence. I simply recorded his country of birth and any more recent travel and moved on.

His reaction to what was an innocent, if perhaps slightly poorly phrased question might be labelled by some as oversensitive. This would miss the point – in particular, the significance of the word 'sensitivity'. In medicine, this word has meaning. Whenever a test to detect something is used, we have to decide how 'sensitive' to make it, how low to set the bar for a positive result, and this is always a trade-off. Lowering the threshold, making it more likely to detect a disease, also makes it more likely you'll get false positives.

This is a concept the US military realised when developing radar. If it's not sensitive enough, you won't spot the bomber before it descends out of the clouds. Make it too sensitive on the other hand, and you'll spend all of your time chasing and machine-gunning flocks of geese you mistook for deadly adversaries.

The same goes for detecting racism as a member of a minority community in the UK – if your awareness is adequately dialled up to detect every time someone is calling you a dickhead to your face, inevitably you'll occasionally think the worst when someone is just asking you about your medical history.

CHAPTER 4

Locks Up Your Hair

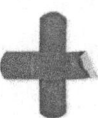

THE REMAINDER OF my FY2 year bled straight into what came next. My job as an SHO on the acute general medicine ward at the Citadel finished on the 5th of August and was immediately followed by another four months of . . . exactly the same. This time, however, in the process of grasping the next rung, I had defected to the rival school across town. Still a teaching hospital that was equally, if not more, steeped in history, a Magisterium of the arcane traditions of medicine – only one whose students and doctors my classmates had sung graphic, unquestionably cancellable (if anatomically accurate) rugby songs about.

Before I left, on hearing I had landed a job there, one of the more jovially antagonistic acute-medicine consultants asked with (I hope) mock incredulity: 'Dr Hutchinson, how did *you* get a job at the Magisterium!?'

'I dunno . . . luck, and bribery.'

General medicine, still an aspect of working in most medical jobs, is an overladen beast of burden. Despite this – the chaotic ward cover, the drowning in acute takes and enduring excruciating post-take ward rounds – I had chosen to enter Core Medical Training (CMT), the two-year staging point for a career in one of the specialties which would guarantee more of the same as I moved through the rotations.[2]

I had gone through university assuming I wanted to be a surgeon, but had found I was more suited to never-ending ward rounds, consumed with tinkering with the numbers, and clinics, which at their worst ranged from the tedious to the unbearably frantic.

The conditions and diagnostic challenges I found interesting were all dealt with by medics. Plus, I lack the attention span for surgery. It felt like operations could go on forever, hours desperate to scratch your nose, suddenly screamingly itchy as soon as the gloves are on. Also, it turns out surgical training is often as much about standing for hours holding a retractor for some operating theatre dictator (benevolent or otherwise) and polishing the teacher's apple as it is moments of glory. And getting scrubbed is a real faff.

On graduating, Louise had been flung out into the wilds of south London. None of her medical school friends had landed in the same patch, so yet again, in need of a flatmate, she turned elsewhere – and found herself lodging in the spare room of Josh, one of my manchild friends from back home. This suited me fine, but meant she had to contend with cleaning that happened biannually at best unless she did it, while he was lying beached on the sofa every Sunday, wallowing in the effects of another Saturday night out.

---

2   This has since been rebranded Integrated Medical Training or 'IMT', with an extra year tacked on just for funzies.

'I can't . . . move . . .'

'Well, perhaps you could try drinking a bit less next time?'

'What, like some kind of melt!?'

We also had to witness his truly bizarre diet. Food was about quantity, no thought to what might be complementary. It wasn't unheard of for him to supplement a meal of spaghetti Bolognese with a side of two salmon fillets. At least Louise had her own bathroom.

The reality of two junior doctor rotas meant there would be weeks where we barely saw one another. Even if we were theoretically sleeping in the same place, night shifts and long days overlapping meant one of us could be leaving while the other was still at work.

Occasionally in medicine, a level of fatigue sets in that stumbles into drunkenness. Thinking is sluggish and meandering, complemented by an over-caffeinated nausea. One CMT job in particular (in a specialty that will remain nameless) reached these heights, its rota containing patterns that were a relic of a bygone era, when doctors lived in the hospital.

The worst I got during that rotation was seven-day blocks of 13-hour shifts in a row, 91 hours in a week (these could be days or nights), bookended by an hour and twenty-minute public transport odyssey across London (no change there). One poor soul however, landed in the slot that, unthinkably, managed to be even worse. When I arrived for the night-time handover, after her 12th straight long day, Alice, normally the most together among us, was so far gone I'm not sure I'd have trusted her to make a cup of tea, let alone touch a patient.

'Mr Sethi in bed five . . . still . . . offloading with IV furosemide . . . I think?' Her usual assured Cardiff accent had been infused with doubt.

'I think you'd better go home. Is anyone about to drop dead, or need anything urgent?'

'No . . .'

'Then I'll figure it out.'

There is abundant evidence that tired people make mistakes. For example, in one experiment, prolonged wakefulness (admittedly for 24 hours) produced the same effect during a psychomotor task as having a blood alcohol of 0.10, above the legal driving limit, which is a problem when said snafu runs the risk of being fatal. This is something the airline industry cottoned on to, and has taken steps to avoid, it being bad for business having planes dropping out of the sky. Medical mishaps, despite also being catastrophic, often remain better hidden among the general messiness of human physiology and frailty. Death is sometimes an inevitability in our line of work. For this reason, although admittedly things aren't quite as bad as they used to be, overwork and fatigue among doctors and other staff has never been addressed satisfactorily. Plus, there already aren't enough doctors, so tough.

Much of our cohort would eventually go on to develop what the registrars called 'CMT syndrome' – extreme frustration and ennui, at knowing enough medicine to be expected to get things right, but being junior enough for the gravity of the hierarchical tract to still deposit the shittiest of tasks on your plate.

The final months of the programme in particular, often spent on jobs that, while important, had little to do with our no doubt glittering future careers, were spent rope-a-doping – waiting for the bell that would signal the end of the slog and the start of registrar training in a specialty we were actually interested in.

* * *

It's a sign of dissatisfaction at work when, on your way in, you are daydreaming about the least severe injury or illness that would still be a viable reason to call in sick. Hit by a car? Maybe a little drastic. A touch of diarrhoea and vomiting from Josh's takeaway leftovers maturing at the back of the fridge, on the other hand? Unpleasant, perhaps, but the 48-hour window after it finished, before you're allowed anywhere near the hospital, would be bliss.

Unfortunately, no such luck. I was back on medical ward cover nights in what passes for fine health. I was now at the stage where I felt confident managing most of what a shift could throw up, but the potential catastrophe in front of me was one where I needed backup from someone older, wiser – and who would make a reliable witness in court if everything really went sour.

'You're not going to poison me like some lab rat!'

'Rob, we just want to help.'

'Leave me alone!'

He had barricaded himself in a corner of the ward corridor, hiding amid a mess of chairs and wielding a drip stand. Michelle and I stood a good five metres back, trying to work out what to do. A reversal of the norm, this 6 ft 3 skinhead was apparently petrified of what I and a 5 ft 2 Chinese-Singaporean woman were about to do to him. Perhaps stripped of his Stone Island jacket, and instead flapping about in a gown, he felt a little vulnerable.

To be fair, one of us (Michelle) *was* holding a syringe full of sleepy juice. Not that you ever want to have to sedate someone, but when it seems possible, or even likely, that a patient may kick someone's head in, it helps to come prepared, just in case. (In an emergency, please be sure to read your trust's easily located and digested rapid tranquillisation protocol.) It was probably false reassurance anyway, as how we ever could have brought down this rhino of a man without a dart gun, I'm not sure.

We also couldn't just leave him there. Aside from the unsightliness of a raging, psychotic giant hiding in a den in the corner of the ward when the bosses came round in the morning, there was the possibility that he might actually be sick. A smoker, he had come in with breathing difficulties – and the level of CO_2 in his blood was high, which by itself is already a problem (as *very* high levels have the inconvenient effect of being fatal). It could also have been contributing to him suddenly behaving erratically, as could the steroids he had been given in ED, coupled with his long history of mental health problems, including psychosis and alcohol dependence.

So, we were left with an agitated man mountain, thinking we were out to kill him, but who needed to be calmed down to allow us to strap a mask to his face to 'help him breathe' – something that some evil scientist *actually* trying to kill him almost certainly might try to do.

Security were on their way, but what they would do when they got there I'm not sure. Before that could be answered, Rob vaulted the barrier and padded down the corridor. His options were limited, since the door out of the ward was closed, and the whole space was one giant square wrapped around the central pillar and nurse's station, so as we followed him it became a sort of bare-cheeked hospital Pac-Man.

Whenever we approached, he would back off, scampering away into the gloom. This would alternate with apparent flashes of awareness of the size imbalance – and he would about-turn and edge towards us. Having silently agreed that neither of us was being paid enough to be hospitalised ourselves, Michelle and I would retreat whenever this happened.

After several slow interminable minutes of this game, the beep and clunk of the automatic doors interrupted. The cavalry was here, having cantered, rather than galloped, up from ED. Unfortunately, Rob was standing nearby and seized this opportunity to expand the playing field. He rushed through the double doors and found himself out in the hallway between wards. This was less than ideal, but at least thanks to the terrible signage, the chances of him finding the stairs in his delirious state were pretty low.

Other than acting as another body to stand in his way, it's not clear what security could offer in this situation. He was big enough that, even with two of them, you wouldn't want to bet on their chances. Besides, Ibrahim and Pavel, as their name badges informed me, seemed to have come to a similar conclusion to us regarding the pay vs lasting physical injury equation. So, they were reduced to hovering in the vicinity, thumbs tucked passively into their stab vests, waiting for something to happen.

It could have been the shift in numbers, perhaps boredom, or maybe he was just tired, but he stopped pacing and sat on one of the banks of chairs lining the wall outside the ward. He hung his head, panting like a stuck buffalo. It was at this point Michelle and I racked our brains, trying to access any scraps we could remember from the conflict resolution and de-escalation e-learning, which, like all NHS staff, we had both clicked through without reading. Am I supposed to keep my hands up or down? Palms open or closed? Remain expressionless, or contort my face into an insincere and creepy grin?

Michelle gave up on pondering this and headed over, syringe now nowhere to be seen.

'Stay away from me. I'm warning you!'

'Fine, I won't come any closer – but you look tired. How about we at least go back to your bed?'

'So you can kill me?'

'No one's going to kill you.'

Then, suddenly channelling a boarding school matron: 'But it's three o'clock in the morning, people are sleeping, and this is all making a *lot* of noise.'

He sat for a while pondering, not saying anything. Then, as if mental as well as physical regression to a childlike state had taken hold, he staggered to his feet and obediently headed back into the ward and his bed. This was of course only a partial victory – we weren't about to high-five one another and send security on their way. We also weren't about to press our luck and a Non-Invasive Ventilation mask onto his face just yet – although we'd have to bite that bullet at some point soon, as it was the only thing that would fix his CO_2 levels.

All the while this had been happening, the stream of patients into ED will have continued, without the rationalising input of the medical SpR allocating doctors to see them and deflecting a few home. Michelle would be lucky if she didn't return to a department jammed up like Greek holiday resort plumbing after some renegade flushing (google it). So, with Rob now back in bed, she began making noises that indicated she would be leaving.

'So just get the nurses to check on him every 15 minutes – and if he falls asleep, whack the mask on him.'

'Whack the mask on him? What if he wakes up and whacks me?'

'Well, then you'll know he's not in a coma.'

This was physiologically accurate at least – the ability to reach out and slap you intentionally relies on a baseline level of consciousness. It's probably equivalent to a 5 or 6 on the 'movement' section of the Glasgow Coma Scale (GCS). For now, anyway, he was still very much awake. He had been led back to bed and appeared to be staying there – but there didn't seem to be any imminent risk of him nodding off. He was hunched under his reading light, eyes scanning the room for potential syringe-wielding assassins.

I hung around for a diplomatic five minutes or so, before deciding it was time to make my own excuses. 'Okay, so Michelle has asked if you could check on him every 15 minutes – and call me if he falls asleep, or if he tries to kill anyone again.'

'And where are *you* going to be?' said Loretta, the ward sister.

Her tone perfectly mixed exasperation at her lot and consternation at what felt like doctors' uncanny ability to disappear at (in)convenient moments, leaving the nurses holding the 100-kilo baby.

She was one of the nurses who knew me best – a Jamaican woman in her late forties, who, on meeting me the first time, before even introducing herself, had asked: 'Hmmm . . . so you locks up ya hair?' Establishing the tone of our relationship, this was delivered maternally, sitting somewhere between affection, respect and patronising – acknowledging what she saw as an effort to engage with my roots, but with the implication I had got a long way to go. At the time, I had cut it relatively short, making it appear as if I was just embarking in baby steps on a natural hair journey.

Predicting what any Jamaican above a certain age, particularly those that would consider themselves respectable, thinks of hair styled in locks is always hard – given the association with Rastafarianism, and the outcast status endured by followers for much of the 20th century. Anyone who looked like they were even flirting with the idea would be viewed with suspicion by good upstanding Christian members of society – worried they were no doubt layabouts ready to commit a crime, or spark up a spliff at a moment's notice. My uncle Alf was so afraid of the response that Vads, the aunt who raised him, would have to his hair, that before one trip home to Jamaica, he resorted to shaving his dreads (a term he uses, but I understand others are less comfortable with) off, rather than face her judgement.

There was something imprinted, something about Loretta's voice and attitude, that meant I was even more inclined to do what I could to stay on her good side. I lived in anxiety over her judgement.

'I have this long list of patients I need to review,' I whined, trying to muster my most authoritative voice, while by way of evidence producing the bundle of ragged sheets of A4 – folded into eighths and scrawled with the initials, hospital numbers and problems of the unfortunates who needed my attention, as was customary. On this occasion this seemed to be sufficient, and I escaped without much more in the way of protest. Thankfully, Rob didn't try to kill anyone else, at least not while I was on shift.

* * *

From the moment I contemplated growing my hair, it has been commented on by what feels like everyone, and has been an issue for some. My secondary school was so white, as soon as I looked like I was entertaining the idea of anything longer than a No. 3 from the clippers, the head of year called me in to a one-on-one meeting. The leadership team were anxious about the apparently (in their minds at least) well-established black-hairstyle-to-knife-crime pipeline.

'Are you planning on putting plaits in your hair?'

'Do you mean cane rows?'

'Any of *that* sort of thing – we'd really rather you didn't.'

'Okay . . . but are they against the uniform policy?'

This was clearly a tricky one; technically they weren't. As a boys' school with this demographic makeup, it hadn't even crossed their minds when writing the rules that this possibility might arise. They could hardly claim cane rows weren't neat – all precise geometric patterns and straight lines. The closest restriction they could find was the need to keep hair shorter than your collar, but that still left far more leeway than they were comfortable with.

'No . . . there isn't an *official* rule against them.'

His voice was heavy with the lament that they couldn't instate an outright ban without appearing overtly, rather than covertly, racist (which had been serving them just fine until now).

The meeting ended without the resolution he hoped for – that my track record as a line-toeing nerd up to this point meant he could rely on my fear of authority and obedience. On the other hand, this unblotted copy book, combined with the fact I wasn't breaking any actual rules, meant there wasn't anything they could do to stop me.

As my hair was growing, before it was long enough to braid, the short afro was a curiosity. Not all of the attention was welcome. On occasion, sitting too close to the reprobates at the back of the class, I'd have to be vigilant to avoid pencils being wedged in, risking my retaliation, which would then mean escalation – a reminder that school is a high-pressured office job, with the added stress you might get punched in the face during your lunch break.

The more significant obstacle to me braiding my hair was financial. As the customers of any salon will tell you, if you can't find a skilled and helpful family member or friend willing to work for free, prepare to pay. Having two boys meant that, up until now, this was one of the cultural exchanges my mother had been able to skip, and she hardly had the time or the means to learn to do it herself now. Eventually, a solution presented itself. A colleague of hers had a side hustle, at a time before the term had been invented. Every other Saturday I'd sit in her living room, my hair being yanked and tightened into whatever pattern MTV Base had implanted in my mind that week, in front of *Soccer AM* (her choice not mine).

The emphasis, here, is definitely on the word 'tightened', because even without the overheads of a shop, and presumably VAT, the price she charged meant we couldn't afford to get it done more frequently. So to make sure the braids lasted the distance, the hair was pulled back until my forehead was stretched with agonising, facelift-like tension. The pain that goes into black hair styling is so extreme, from tightening, to chemical relaxers, that I maintain the average regular salon client could teach the SAS a thing or two about holding out against interrogation and torture.

Since these less informed times of 'back in my day', the issue of black hair in schools has been more definitively tested. Schools attempting to exclude children on the basis of supposedly unsuitable hairstyles have faced the ire of empowered parents.

That isn't to say it doesn't still happen; it most certainly does, but the issue is being talked about, and the Equality and Human Rights Commission have issued specific guidance, warning schools against policies that don't make allowances for racial differences in hairstyle.

In 2020, pupil Ruby Williams received an out-of-court settlement of £8,500 from her school. This was after years of being singled out, having been told her afro hair risked blocking the view of the board for other pupils, which sounds like a lazy sight gag from some terrible comedy script. Other schools have faced protests for banning natural hairstyles, including locks, and have been forced to back down.

What once may have been perceived as 'exotic', and even unprofessional, has become more acceptable in the most establishment bastions in the land. It's misguided to believe a person's beliefs will be formed exclusively according to their race, and also understandable to not want to be defined by it, but the irony is not lost on me of Kemi Badenoch, leading the opposition in the Houses of Parliament, waging the 'war on woke' from the dispatch box in braids. That hairstyle in that place has become normalised in no small part thanks to the spilled blood of many a social justice warrior, martyred in their existential struggle against microaggressions.

In the 90s, at my Lewisham primary school, on the other hand, I had faced almost the inverse issue – trying to keep up with the styles on the playground was the struggle. I must have been around six when I convinced my parents it wasn't going to be viable for them to go on cutting my hair themselves if I wanted to escape school without PTSD, and they finally took me to a barber.

Every clipper gradient was a battle and a negotiation with my dad – 'No, you can't have a No. 1 all over, but yes, if you really have to, you can shave a Nike tick into the back of your head . . .' The same all-out consumerism that dominated the shoe game on the playground was being etched into the boys' scalps, and I didn't want to be left out. They drew the line at three stripes in the eyebrows, however. The crowning moment in my junior hair odyssey was the high-top fade – a look I was rocking arguably long after peak popularity, and deep into the mid-1990s. By the time I gave the look up, *The Fresh Prince of Bel Air* had aired its final episode.

The site of this salvation, 'First Glance' in Brockley, is still there. It's a well-worn trope, but a true one, that a barber shop serves far more of a purpose than simply cutting hair. It can be community centre, social club and business networking hub – as immortalised in the black British comedy classic *Desmond's*. The barber shop was the first place I can remember hearing Kiss and Choice FM, the Saturday morning soundtrack to the staff's conversations, alluding to whatever they got up to last night, or what they had planned for that evening in as coded and child-friendly terms as they could manage. In any case, if any of the young barbers were hungover, it never seemed to affect the neatness of the fade.

The role of barber shops in community is not simply some folksy romanticisation, but rather has real significance. This has been recognised by a number of public health initiatives, which have used them to target in-need but difficult-to-reach individuals, disseminating information about type 2 diabetes and hypertension, both in the UK and the US. (I'd like to pitch the tagline 'in the chair, cutting blood pressure, sugar and hair'.)

In the 2002 film of the same name, Cedric the Entertainer describes the barber shop as 'our country club' – and it is that, but much more besides. As a sounding board, while the customer is in the chair, barbers and hairdressers may well be the longest conversation a person has all week. Willingly or otherwise, they can find themselves as much a therapist as a stylist – the chair metamorphosising into a couch. They can be well placed to see that a person is struggling with their mental health, and this has been formalised with initiatives offering formal training for barbers, through schemes such as 'the Barbers Project' in Islington, specifically targeting black men.

* * *

At university, among medical students, my hair (now bound up in locks) was such a point of difference that it was enough for people to just say 'dreads' to know who they were talking about. For much of my time at medical school, no one else among the 2,500 or so of us that made up all six years would have fit the description. Not that I particularly minded – any negative impact of this form of exoticism is often not felt in the moment. Much better to be recognisable for something than nothing.

My parents had been given the well-meaning warning by a friend who used to lecture at the medical school that my hair might hold me back – and perhaps it has, in ways that remain hidden and I'll never see. Points may have been knocked off an interview, or a poor first impression with a new boss, our relationship soured before I've even had a chance to earn their disdain with any incompetence. But no one in a position of power has ever instructed me to get a haircut – and I personally can be pretty satisfied with how my career in medicine has panned out.

This wasn't a guarantee. Some consultant surgeons, operating theatre autocrats, were known to dictate the length of hair and shaving habits of even their privately educated white male underlings, regardless of whether tucked away safely during operations. (There even exists such a thing as a 'beard snood' for the maintenance of hygiene, an image that will haunt your dreams if you google it.) So, if apex privilege doesn't get you a pass, it's hardly a stretch to imagine them finding fault with something so far from a short back and sides as my hair.

One thing that may have spared me this particular battle with the higher-ups is my aforementioned tendency to avoid surgeons and theatre whenever possible. I can count on one hand the number of times I have crammed my hair under a cap and stood there, bored, since graduating. It's also possible that, having seen other organisations burned in the past, hospital management have decided it's just not worth their while.

Unequal treatment of employees with black and natural hairstyle does still remain an issue in a wide range of professions. Attitudes of bosses and other decision-makers can act as a barrier to progression – the World Afro Hair Day organisation commissioned the 'World Hair Acceptance Report', which included a survey of 1,000 employers and found marked differences in the acceptance of Eurocentric compared to afro styles.

The report also highlighted the case of Jerelle Jules, who, in the process of applying for a job at the Ritz, was sent an employee grooming policy banning 'unusual hairstyles', including 'afro style'. There can be little as outright othering as an employer plainly stating that the most basic description of your hair as it grows naturally is considered 'unusual' and prohibited. The Ritz claimed he had been sent an out-of-date policy (no arguments there). A British establishment institution behaving in this manner, however, is emblematic of what many black people rightly suspect is the attitude towards them and their appearance in these places.

* * *

Back on days, I had been asked to come down from the ward and help in clinic, as one of the rheumatology SpRs who normally did the list had done the unthinkable and called in sick (the lucky so-and-so). Given my limited specialty experience at the time, it was hardly a like-for-like swap for the patient who would be seeing me instead, but in any case, lupus clinics are often an all-hands-on-deck affair. If patients really need to be seen, then they are, even if the clinic is already 100 per cent overbooked. On busy days, the waiting room can look like the fallout from some disaster – bodies on every surface, or crowding the desk, clamouring for attention from reception staff.

'Have you had any hair loss?' is a question that might not be the first thing you expect your doctor to be fixated on when assessing you for a potentially life-threatening disease, but in rheumatology, we ask almost everyone. Lupus can affect any part of the body, including the follicles. It might seem superficial to worry about your hair and skin when a disease is destroying your kidneys, but renal failure doesn't have people double-taking when you walk past them on the street.

Hair loss can be distressing for anyone – but clearly, because of the burdens imposed by society, it's often a particular issue for women. Losing it in clumps, and often with angry red rashes where the hair has fallen out, is enough to leave many patients tearful and desperate.

Owing to the differences in how hair grows (it can be slower even once lupus has been brought back under control), and the aforementioned products and regimens, the effect on black hair can be particularly damaging. Fixing braided extensions when there are huge gaps in the places you would normally anchor them is rarely going to yield the desired result.

It's part of developing, maturing as a doctor (hopefully), learning to take seriously the things like this that matter to patients.

'My hair? It all gone . . . long time ago.' In her Congolese accent, she said this with what might be taken as unexpected, even inappropriate lightness, smiling, almost laughing. But at this point the team had grown accustomed to her navigating the most harrowing spells of her disease with an amused detachment, at times seemingly floating above them as if they were happening to someone else.

Every few years, her immune system seemed to get bored – waking from a slumber to have another go at trying to kill her. Kidney failure, myocarditis, gut inflammation – she had weathered it all, seemingly indestructible.

She pointed to the violet silk wrap covering her head, and then pinched some of the strands of braided hair that protruded from underneath.

'It's a wig . . . it all fake!'

She laughed again, and it was hard to know if this was at my naivety, having been fooled by the hairpiece, or because she had by this point been through so much that all of our questions, suggesting we might have any real insight, some ability to predict when she was becoming more unwell by consulting the medical tea leaves, seemed faintly absurd. Fortunately, however, for both of us, her illness was very much in its dormant phase. The primary purpose of that day's appointment seemed to be humouring me and my belief that I had the ability to change things.

Much like the experience of patients with cancer after chemotherapy, lupus-related hair loss can become so severe that the only option becomes a wig. Depending on what you can afford, these can range from the unconvincing, spotted-from-a-mile-off variety, to luxurious yet undetectable works of art. Some funding is available, but the NHS is unfortunately unlikely to cover the cost of a follicular Rolls-Royce, making this yet another financial burden of being unwell. For those who choose for their hair extensions and replacements to match their natural hair texture, there has also historically been difficulty obtaining products derived from donated afro hair.

Despite all I've said, hair loss in lupus, and the resulting need for hair coverings and wigs, is, paradoxically, one of the few disease domains where (in one specific way) some black patients are perhaps closer to a level playing field. Without wishing to oversimplify a deeply sensitive and often contentious issue, many black people in the UK choose to wear wigs, even in the absence of any illness affecting their hair – meaning that, should the need arise, the transition may be less noticeable and provoke less self-consciousness.

The same can't be said for the often-accompanying myriad skin symptoms that are also hallmarks of this disease. Skin inflammation leading to loss of pigment and abnormal healing (including the development of 'keloid' scars) is frequently more noticeable and severe in darker skin. Open any course-recommended medical textbook used in the US and UK, and one thing is abundantly clear. The majority of the skin on display in the myriad pictures of illnesses is white. On the surface, this may not be much of a surprise – these books are being authored in countries with majority white populations, and when the statistics are reviewed, some do in fact represent the US population according to racialised ethnic group.

Looking a little deeper, however, a problem emerges. Even among those ethnic minority group images used, the vast majority of skin tone on display is light. The Massey–Martin skin score grades skin from 1 (very light) to 10 (very dark). While acknowledging it is far from perfect (a scale designed to grade skin tones – what could be problematic about that?), using this tool, authors found that dark skin representation was as low as 0.31 per cent in one textbook, as compared to the US population proportion of 11 per cent. Other books were admittedly less skewed, ranging from 1.1 per cent to 8.4 per cent.

This has the potential to cause real harm – to lead to delayed diagnosis. Without wishing to dent the prices my esteemed colleagues are able to charge for private work, dermatology is often a 'say what you see' exercise. In order to do this, medical students and doctors need to be given the tools to recognise rashes and the other skin manifestations of disease – in all of the skin types that may present to them. It is increasingly recognised that even common skin complaints such as eczema and psoriasis can present 'atypically' (by the standards of Eurocentric medicine) in darker skin. This is a personal experience recounted by Dr Layal Liverpool in her book *Systemic*.

The danger of this disparity is exported and compounded by the dominance of medical literature and research coming out of Europe and America. Even in countries with global majority, non-white populations, it is often likely that healthcare staff are trained using materials from these systems, with a knock-on effect on care.

The effects of skin tone on the provision of care are another ingredient added to the formulation of injustices experienced by people on the basis of their darker skin – the global tendency for those with darker skin tones to face more discrimination and be granted fewer opportunities. Colourism is a colonial leftover that can lead to a gradient in social hierarchies and the popularity of 'remedies' such as dangerous skin-lightening products, which remain depressingly popular worldwide, their use continuing to cause damage.

In an effort to right this imbalance, motivated individuals have taken steps – including enviably precocious medical students such as Malone Mukwende, who authored the textbook *Mind the Gap*, a resource showing clinical signs in darker skin tones, while still studying at St George's. Naabil Khan set up the website 'Skin For All' with similar intentions while at university in Exeter (the hustle spirit is clearly strong in Gen-Z; I'll soon be out of a job unless I'm careful). What remains, however, is for these materials to be made a standard part of mainstream medical education.

CHAPTER 5

In the Blood

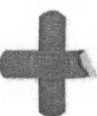

THE OXYGEN MASK was gripped in his left hand, and he held the bed frame with the other. He breathed deeply and deliberately, eyes closed, as if engaged in some excruciating meditation.

I was now at a hospital that if you're keen on the well-worn 'frontline' metaphor, would best be described as 'the Trench'. It was the local hospital for a larger area of more deprived, more unwell patients. Plugging these bits of data into the equation dictating how much work there is for the acute teams to do, the result = too much. It was one of the placements trainees discussed in hushed tones.

'Oh, you're going *there* next? Good luck . . .'

The kind of medicine that puts hair on your chest as an SHO, calluses on your hands, and makes anywhere you go afterwards seem tame by comparison.

Haematology patients were our responsibility out of hours. Whenever a 'red cell' admission landed, the call came straight to me. People (other doctors included) don't realise, but far from being sedate, blood disorders are another specialty that can serve up a barrage of chaos, emergencies and heartache.

Tribal tattoos wrapped from his deltoids to his forearms. Between the ink spirals, the skin was darker than mine, but not by much.

Lacking the funds to clamber out of the Dark Ages into the bright NHS digital future, the ED were still clinging resolutely to their paper notes and drug charts. Before I could do anything, I would need to go on a frantic scavenger hunt to find them and check what he had already been given and to write up the something stronger he clearly needed.

'How are you doing, Theo?'

Despite the pain, he was still sufficiently present to acknowledge the inanity of the question, opening his eyes and meeting my gaze with his own – one that asked: 'How does it look like it's going?'

'Not . . . great . . .'

The emphasis lent by the pauses nailed home the point.

Fingers possessed by nervous energy, I awkwardly spun the head of my stethoscope from the diaphragm to the bell position and back again, clicking with each movement. 'Yes, sorry – let me just go and get your drug chart.'

I ducked out and headed desperately to the numbered slots. The chances of finding a patient's notes where they were supposed to be during peak hours was minimal. Time-pressed doctors and nurses tidied away like six-year-olds at the end of play, stuffing paper bundles into any crack or crevice that kept them out of sight. You were almost as likely to find a half-eaten sandwich or browning banana tucked away as the file you were looking for. Miraculously, however, when I looked, his CAS card was sitting neatly waiting for me.

Paracetamol, oramorph – not nothing, but clearly not enough. Fortunately, as with many serious conditions presenting to the ED, there is a sickle cell protocol endorsing liberal prescribing (in theory). Equally important at this moment, there was a free and functioning computer that meant I could print it out.

I returned to his room, if not triumphant, then at least confident I could now be of some use.

'Does subcut morphine normally work for you?'

'You can try . . . but I think I need a PCA.'

Caught out again. Patient-controlled anaesthesia allows them to take charge of their own relief, delivering it at the touch of a button – meaning they don't need to rely on the divided attentions of nursing staff. The downside: hanging up a bag of potentially lethal drugs safely is a specialist skill.

I found the nurse looking after him to at least give him something, before heading to the phone to negotiate with anaesthetics.

* * *

Sickle cell is a genetic disease causing red blood cells to distort under certain conditions like cold and during infections, getting stuck in blood vessels, causing excruciating pain and risking severe organ damage. The condition overwhelmingly affects people with African ancestry, and it should be no surprise that this has impacted the experience of sufferers. It isn't a ringing endorsement of our past practice as a profession that we need a cheat sheet to remind us to do our jobs and provide adequate pain relief. But apparently that's what it takes – historically, analgesia during sickle crises has been variable, with staff sometimes slow to prescribe the good stuff and, in some cases, not giving it at all.

In the UK, recent audits have shown poor performance

persists – the majority of centres in the UK for which data are available fail to meet the NICE target of delivering treatment to these patients within 30 minutes of presentation to A&E.

As with everything, the reasons behind this are complex. If we're being charitable to our medical ancestors, even in patients with severe pain from sickle cell, outwardly there can be very little revealing how unwell they really are (of course, other than them *telling* you they feel terrible).

Race also undoubtedly also plays a role. The story of the treatment of sickle cell by Western healthcare systems is punctuated by dismissal of patients as melodramatic, malingering or drug-seeking.

Patients often know what works for them, given they have experienced these episodes since childhood. Admittedly, most people who come through the door asserting that diamorphine (aka heroin) is what they need should probably be treated with at least some caution, maybe asked a few follow-up questions, but that's why specific knowledge is needed. Levels of understanding among doctors and, with it, willingness to prescribe is linked to the disease prevalence in an area.

Running counter to the rationing going on with sickle patients in the ED, during my time at medical school we were still being taught that addiction in patients given these drugs for medical reasons almost never happened (this is a paradox which was never reconciled, and with prejudice no doubt playing a major role in this disparity). In any case, a little digging by the first journalist who bothered to look exposed the shaky matchstick foundations of this idea.

The often quoted 'study' reporting extremely low rates of dependence in the context of opioid use in a range of diseases was just a letter to the editor of the *New England Journal of Medicine* –

a physician relaying his uncontrolled observations from a single US hospital. The word of one single good old boy leading to purely vibes-based international medical dogma and teaching, passed down as gospel through the years.

Among patients exposed to opioids for any condition, for prolonged periods of time, a minority *will* develop issues with addiction. The devastation of the opioid crisis in the US has demonstrated this, with sports injuries and back pain becoming the first limping steps on the path to addiction, and in some cases destitution or even death.

There is no evidence that patients with sickle cell are any more at risk than comparable groups given these medications – although as with other aspects of the disease, it is understudied. And if we are so worried about the risks of addiction and drug-seeking behaviour among this population, where are the services to help prevent it?

Acknowledging the existence of dependence, while arguing for more liberal use of pain relief may sound like a contradiction. But the net effect of the accepted approach has been to withhold adequate pain relief in the short term from sickle patients who need it, while also failing to adequately manage dependence in the minority over the long term when it does develop.

In any case, this dependence would be less likely with better long-term management of sickle cell disease itself – reducing the frequency of painful crises requiring these drugs. And management does need to be better – research into new therapies has historically been underfunded, as are the NHS services that deliver them.

Until recently, management was mainly limited to avoiding activities and environments likely to trigger crises, and a medi-cation called hydroxycarbamide – which can reduce the frequency by around 50 per cent, but isn't without side effects. Red cell exchanges, which are exactly what they sound like – a switcheroo, where sickling blood is swapped out during a crisis – are also used. But this carries the dual issues of having to sit in hospital, and the risks associated with repeated blood transfusions. Bone marrow transplants are in theory an option, but carry the undesirable side effect of a significant risk of death (7 per cent in one study).

In the last few years, the *Tomorrow's World* sci-fi technology of CRISPR gene editing has bucked the trend of neglect, and yielded the closest thing to a cure. The poisoned incentives of the pharmaceutical industry being what they are, however, the drug is so expensive (in the region of £1.5 million per patient for a one-off course) you could set the vial in a ring and wear it as jewellery to rival the Crown Jewels. Predictably, there has been a fight with NICE, although the treatment has finally been approved.

The disease isn't abstract or totally alien to me. I had an aunt with the condition, and I still have a cousin. I am a carrier, with the 'trait', which means under most circumstances, too few of my cells are liable to go rogue to cause much of a problem. There is a risk at extremes of atmospheric pressure, meaning my dreams of glittering mountaineering and scuba careers have been cruelly ended before they even started. It hardly has a major direct impact on my life, though it is a reminder of a shared heritage, that others linked to me have been less fortunate.

It's rarely a good look when advocates for one disease or service pit themselves against another, highlighting differences in resources or attention. With sickle cell, however, there has always been the temptation to look at another genetic condition, one with a similar (although actually lower) prevalence in the UK and US, with similar life-restricting capacity, but admittedly a greater impact on longevity.

Cystic fibrosis can often seem like the inverted white negative image, seeing as that's the group most likely to be affected. The two have long been compared, with the feeling that cystic fibrosis is the favoured child, receiving more attention, empathy and the all-important bottom line: money. Over the years, estimates of the disparity have varied, depending on the context, but for example in the US, in 2011, National Institute for Health funding per affected person was 11 times higher for cystic fibrosis. The belief being that if white people got sickle cell, it would receive more of everything. While this may be true, comparing diseases like this overlooks that these people are all suffering.

A young patient I will never forget was playing five-a-side right up until the week she came into hospital, living life to the full despite the toll cystic fibrosis had taken. She was admitted with another infection; these can be the stepwise knocks that cause lungs to fail. But even in hospital her spirit and resilience gave me pause to reflect.

Realising she may be in for a while, her family had brought in a guitar, and the sounds of her (mercifully adept) playing echoed through the corridors, soundtracking my evenings on call – haunting (mainly instrumental) John Lewis Christmas advert-style reimaginings of classic pop songs. Even now, I can't hear Luther Vandross's 'Never Too Much' without thinking of that time.

She had been in so many times before, enduring the miserable routine of chest-pummelling physiotherapy and the interminable wait for the IV antibiotics to work. So, when this time they didn't, it blindsided everyone – her, her family, and the team looking after her.

This memory means I won't scapegoat one disease for the sake of another. It is, however, important that we treat these two comparable conditions with the equity that is deserved – bringing sickle cell up to parity, and ultimately just doing better for both.

* * *

The haematology ward, where the sickle cell patients land, can take on an atmosphere that feels alien in comparison to others. If enough are in together, the average age plummets. When you cohort people in their late teens and twenties together, the dynamics have more in common with a youth club than a place for the ill and infirm.

That isn't to say they don't need to be there – they're all sick, it's just that when these admissions become the norm, life goes on. Friendships form and break among the 'frequent flyers', arguments over who's too loud, who's rude.

'You can't put them next to each other – Janelle *hates* Mercy . . . something about a boy from last time.'

These out-of-hours shifts can drag you between extremes. It had started with a good old-fashioned medical car crash – a woman in her sixties with lymphoma, on chemotherapy, had arrived in the assessment unit downstairs looking less than well.

I had been dimly made aware of her at the handover – that there was a woman the day SHO had seen, but not yet admitted, feeling generally ill, but little else. When I arrived, she was grey, a sign which, in white patients, where these things are visible, is ironically a red flag.

'I just feel . . . so tired.'

A remarkable number of the diagnostic signs and tests in critical illness are founded on the assumption that the patient's skin lacks much in the way of that *oh so inconvenient* melanin – obscuring what's going on underneath. This issue was brought in to focus during the pandemic, when it was pointed out that the

O_2 finger probes, relying on measuring light absorption, might just be affected by colour (screw you, racist physics!). At worst, the trace from some patients may have been as reliable as sticking said finger in the air and guessing.

In keeping with her appearance, when I rechecked them, her numbers were all hovering around the 'FFS' regions of the chart: her heart rate was high, and her blood pressure was low. In an infection, numbers like these are signposts on the road to sepsis and death – which had the effect of sending mine upwards.

Sepsis is not really a complete diagnosis on its own – other than to say there is an infection *somewhere*, it's bad, and your body is overreacting, to the point it might kill you, adopting a scorched-earth policy against the invader. It falls under the category of 'act now, think later' situations – the most important thing is giving antibiotics that will treat almost anything. Once things are under control, you can then get on with the chin-stroking attempts at working out exactly where it is.

'Has she had fluids?'

'Nope.'

'Antibiotics?'

'Ermm . . . also no . . . She does have a cannula though.'

This last detail was almost said by the nurse with the expectation it would be greeted with a gold star for effort.

Chemotherapy is often not a friend to the immune system. In killing the cancerous white blood cells, there had no doubt been plenty of innocent bystanders that went with them. This was confirmed when checking her blood results, which had just trickled in from the lab: the Neutrophil count was 0.4. All you need to know about that number is that it is low – low enough to leave her unprotected.

Fortunately, in medicine, when something is both serious and common, this is another situation when the idiot-proof cheat sheet telling us what to do comes into play. We even get children's TV-worthy mnemonics – 'the sepsis six', a list of life-saving tasks the old man in me can imagine the kids doing a TikTok dance about.

At least she had access, which saved me stabbing hopelessly at her veins – she was dehydrated to the point of dustbowl dry, so they would have been totally collapsed. Next, she needed antibiotics and fluid – a major part of medicine can be boiled down to giving antibiotics, and deciding if a patient needs more or less water in their circulation. In this situation, fortunately the answer was obvious.

Saying you want something to happen, writing it down and then ensuring it actually does are all equally important. The ideal is to witness the drugs being given before disappearing to deal with anything else. At times, however, this is a luxury.

Inevitably, there was a cannula that *did* need doing back up on the ward. Now this is obviously a routine procedure that any doctor fresh out of medical school should be able to do.

I will confess right now, I have never been the best at cannulas – but through hard practice and perseverance, I had finally ascended the dizzying heights of being 'not bad'. I knew where to look for a vein – ideally tethered, back of the hand, downstream of a junction. I had learned to be patient, not rushing in with task-blindness when there was no emergency – all the tricks, gravity, warming up the hand to bring veins to the surface.

Even so, not all lines are inserted equal. Sickle cell patients and their veins have suffered a lifetime of punishment at the shaky hands of doctors and nurses, leaving them with scars – both vascular and psychological.

There's a lot of smug chat from anaesthetists regarding

cannulation, and we all know they are the best at it. But as they like to remind us, they are 'not a cannulation service . . .' Practice, of course, makes perfect – during their training they luxuriate for long periods as supernumerary spare parts on operating lists, just there to learn – one-to-one tuition from learned consultants in the finer points of their procedures. Their practice (I imagine) is soundtracked by the twinkling of classical music from the theatre stereo, and the gentle encouraging cooing of their boss over their shoulder. They seem to forget this quickly, however, assuming instead they were born gifted, the rest of us incompetent, lazy, or both.

With procedures, preparation is key: have everything ready in advance. No one wants to watch you scrabble around looking for stuff. Dry your hands before putting on your gloves, otherwise they'll stick – nothing dents patients' confidence in your skills more than an apparent inability to dress yourself.

I stood outside the curtain.

'Knock knock.'

I instantly regretted the smarm of this.

There was a sigh from the other side.

'Come in then.'

'I'm here to put in a new cannula.'

'Are you good? Because they've been messing up my arms.'

'Sure . . . and either way, I won't keep going if I can't find anything.'

'You're right, you won't! You get one chance.'

She had barely looked up in the time I had been in the room, and the video call on the phone in her lap continued almost uninterrupted.

'The doctor's just here.' I got the sense that whoever was on the other end would get a blow-by-blow review of my performance.

A thread on X (formerly Twitter) took off recently, where commentators weighed in on a white doctor complaining that black patients were often on their phones during consultations, outraged at the supposed rudeness and disrespect. His error was quickly pointed out, shall we say 'enthusiastically', by people who actually either were themselves, or knew the patients he was moaning about. For black patients – or for any marginalised person for that matter – having an advocate present, whether in person or remotely, could mean the difference between being treated properly and having your concerns dismissed. Consciously, or subconsciously, most people, including healthcare staff, are less likely to misbehave when there are witnesses.

If a patient has their friends or family at the end of the phone, rather than being a dick about it, might I suggest simply saying hello to them – as you would if they were in the room?

'Where's normally good?'

Without speaking, she presented her left hand. I had a look. Barely visible, thread-like contours mapped the back of her hand. I set about trying to coax them out, a process that inevitably involves some awkward combination of slapping and stroking, the kind of manhandling that under other circumstances would probably get you arrested.

Eventually, the most promising candidate identified itself. As she said, I'd only get one chance at this. I unsheathed the needle and held my breath.

'Sharp scratch' – the old lie, words repeated so often they feel sacred, bad luck not to incant them.

This time, patience was rewarded and my ego was intact – the saline flush went in smoothly, without a grimace, no ballooning around the vein. There was no need for the 'it's probably in, let me just try and save it' wishful thinking that so often accompanies difficult attempts. Taking no chances, I secured it as if swaddling a screaming newborn and moved to make my escape before anything could go wrong.

'There you go.'

'Thanks' was muttered without looking up.

I headed back to the main walkway that ran the length of the ward. Looking into the male bay opposite, I could see Theo. He was slowly wheeling a drip stand hung with a bag of fluid to the bathroom. Although clearly not completely out of the woods, it was a relief to see him no longer writhing and grimacing.

I raised a hand and gingerly waved. I'm not sure if I was hoping for some rapturous response, being greeted like some long-lost friend, but he answered my gesture with an understated nod that revealed very little, and continued his journey.

CHAPTER 6
My Name Is My Name

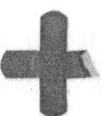

IT HAD BEEN the final CMT job that made up my mind. Excluding specialties from the list of options was like a game of Guess Who?. 'Will I have to learn any difficult equations?' If the answer was 'yes', it was instantly stricken from the list. 'How gross can it get?' . . . that was gastroenterology gone. 'How much shouting can I expect?' I'll leave you to imagine which specialties were crossed off on the basis of that one . . .

Working as an SHO in rheumatology gave me a glimpse of a life I could at least cope with – and, dare to dream, even enjoy. Like the renal doctors, they got to look after patients with the most interesting illnesses – and often make them better. They were spared the maelstrom that can be an inpatient kidney ward, however, the constant threat of someone bleeding torrentially or having a heart attack, always a dialysis catheter needing inserting.

Moving on to the next and final tier of training, becoming a registrar means competing for a 'training number' in your specialty, fighting in a desperate scrum for the rope ladder dangled from the chopper to career safety. Each year, depending on how many senior colleagues are graduating from the pathway, a certain quantity of these will be tossed out. It's the luck of the draw whether you find yourself becoming eligible in a glut or a drought. Doctors aspiring to the most competitive specialties can tread water for years waiting to get in.

I hadn't managed to drive Louise away, despite the more testing elements of my still juvenile late twenties persona (I still slept on a donated futon in a bedroom bereft of any decorations, soft furnishings or even a lampshade). In perhaps a leap of faith, we had decided to skip renting together and instead save to buy somewhere. This meant each of us moving back to the Hotel Parental, so I spent the next months revising for the application in my teenage bedroom, like some wizened A-level student.

I was lucky in terms of the total number of jobs available and the timing of their release. My CV was just about good enough to get me shortlisted, and then the interview (a circuit of stations, a mix of mock clinical scenarios and the good old-fashioned, 'so, tell us why you want to join our club' questions) went smoothly to the point it almost felt perverse.

This is by no means a universal experience for non-white doctors at interview. There is still a clear disparity in terms of the proportion of ethnic minority candidates considered 'appointable' during the medical specialty interview process, compared to their White British counterparts. As much as I'd love to think some innate brilliance allowed me to hurdle towering adversity, in reality all of this will be multifactorial, and I will have been aided by accent, class and colourism.

So there I finally had a concrete answer to the perpetual 'what are you going to be when you grow up?' question, so beloved of smarmy medical elders. I was going to be a rheumatologist, a master of chin-stroking, antibodies and steroids.

* * *

In the hospital, like many young medics, I will more often than not have a stethoscope draped over my shoulders. There is a simple and practical explanation for this: since white coats were banished to the laundry basket in the sky, very few outfits come with pockets large enough to accommodate them.

The accessory is also a rite of passage, however. I can clearly remember fellow medical students proudly unfurling their gleaming 3M Littmanns, names engraved on the bell – the industry standard that the profession has collectively decided is the only acceptable choice, if you don't want to be seen as incompetent, or a weirdo.

It is a statement – one that says what your job is, and, almost as importantly, what it isn't. This can be more vital for some than it is for others. Kyron, a friend from university, and an anaesthetics and intensive care SpR, has on more than one occasion been mistaken for a porter if he wanders around in scrubs without this signifier. Sitting behind a public-facing computer with just my unadorned shirt collar visible, to many visitors I'm clearly the ward clerk.

It may never be enough. Many female doctors I know, despite stethoscope and the full history-taking, clinical assessment and presentation of a diagnosis and plan (and the fact they introduced themselves as 'Doctor'), will finish with a patient, only to be asked: 'Thanks, nurse, now when am I going to see the doctor?'

Before getting too far down this road, a desire not to be mistaken for any of these other roles is indicative of a different problem. It shows how much of a hierarchy still exists – and how those working in them are treated. I'm also well aware that nurse practitioners exist, but they're hardly the default, and probably not what the patient was thinking of.

During my FY1 year in Essex, at one of the weekly teaching sessions designed to fig-leaf the idea that these were training jobs, the consultant taking the session took it upon himself to dispense some pearls on self-confidence and belief coming from within, not a dangling necklace of rubber tubing and a couple of earpieces.

'You guys don't need to walk around with your stethoscopes draped over your necks . . . People will listen to you because of your knowledge and ability.'

Wise words from a tall white guy with a south of England accent, who professionally came of age in the 1980s, well-meant as I'm sure they were.

So, every morning as I stepped into clinic during my ST3 year, as a newly minted rheumatology SpR, alongside the ironed shirt and brogues, the ostentatious gold bell and diaphragm remained on show.

This was likely influenced by the fact that when it came to the finer points of the specialty, what it would take to actually help the person in front of me, it felt like I knew nothing at all. I was also aware that many patients will have been waiting an age for this appointment – so looking the part for first impressions was probably a good idea, an attempt to avoid any 'Six months . . . for this guy!? He can't *really* be the specialist . . .'

* * *

Clinic can in some ways be more stressful than the wards. Sure, you get to sit down, which is a massive plus, but you're the only one responsible for how things are going. Patients arrive expecting to be seen at a specific time. Thirty minutes for a new patient and

15 for a follow-up may sound like plenty, particularly if you're a GP reading this, expected to deal with whatever comes through the door – from a cold to cancer – in 10 minutes. It's never enough, though, and once they're in the room, no one will put up with being yanked offstage by the vaudeville hook before they're ready, just so you can keep to time. Fortunately, I had started out back at the Magisterium – somewhere I had time to think, sharing a list of patients with the consultant, rather than being thrown to the wolves to fend for myself.

Outpatients had recently installed an automated call system. In theory, I pressed a button, and the AI voice, the receptionist of the future, would robotically summon the patient. That day, the success rate had been around 50 per cent; the other times I had to resort to venturing into the corridor to rescue the poor lost wandering souls. I called for the next patient and waited a couple of minutes, before poking my head out of the door. She limped around the corner, each step clearly requiring monumental effort and causing pain. This most likely went some way towards explaining her greeting when she met me at the door.

'Oh God, not another one.'

Not the opening *I'd* go for with the person responsible for my health, but each to their own. 'Another one' could, of course, have multiple meanings, but at this early stage I was willing to give her the benefit of the doubt. I'd presume she was just venting at the prospect of seeing yet another registrar in clinic for the first time, and having to explain her problems over again. A white woman in her sixties, sandy hair scraped into a matronly bun, she had an air of no nonsense, and the boot-and-gilet combination that spoke to mud-flecked Land Rovers and Labradors.

'Hello, Ms Worthing, please come in.'

I have learned over the years of doing clinics that the best way of dealing with the slightest bitter hint of hostility, at first at least, is to douse it in syrup-like obsequiousness. Adopt the air of a hotel concierge, where nothing is too much trouble, service is always delivered with a rictus smile, and after consultation, petit fours delivered with the non-existent bill. This helps me to meet and deflect the patient's perturbed look when they see my lock-framed face. They may even listen to what I have to say if I *really* lay it on thick.

I was prepared for this to be an uphill struggle from the outset anyway – having had the rare luxury of time to properly read her notes between patients. Hers was a problem I was almost certainly unable to solve. Paradoxically in rheumatology, it can be simpler (although not better) for everyone if a patient has some angry, potentially life-threatening immune system disease. It's obvious in their joints, skin and blood tests – and the need for treatment not up for much debate (even if they choose not to take it). Pain without much to see, on the other hand, is much harder.

You're then stuck with being poked and prodded by some well-meaning idiot like me. You grimace and moan in all the right places, but there's nothing to see, the bloods are unexciting, the scans a barren grey wasteland. Clearly there's something wrong, but not anything one of the many shiny immune-system-baffling antibodies we dish out is likely to fix.

This can lead to a frustrating, repetitive cycle – you come in, tell us the same worsening list of symptoms. We look sympathetic (ideally), say there aren't any drugs that will make it better, suggest physiotherapy (which can really work, if you can get it) or, if we're desperate, a steroid injection of questionable utility. Probably fair enough, then, when many of these patients make it clear they think we're useless.

Ms Worthing's problem was her shoulders – but not the kind

of obvious joint damage that might let ortho start revving their drills. Hers was a more subtle nagging from the overstretched and overworked tendons, the musculo-skeletal equivalent of the aforementioned strained NHS GP. In this case, I ended up offering her what some of the more old-school, seasoned consultants would consider a cop out – an ultrasound, with the dual benefit of reassuring everyone there was no inflammation and the chance for an injection all at once.

'In my day, we trusted our examinations,' my superiors may cry – and I'm sure many of them are far better than me when it comes to groping their way to a diagnosis.

Ordering the test had at least convinced her I was doing *something*, taking her seriously – rather than fobbing her off, as patients often assume is a doctor's default position. As I came closer to dragging the consultation to a close, she suddenly perked up, reanimated by some sudden thought.

'Dr Hutchinson, that's a very *British* surname.'

She wasn't technically wrong, but it still didn't feel like there was an appropriate response, other than 'what the fuck do you mean by that?', but I didn't think my professional standing was sturdy enough yet to take the hit.

'Right, yes, I suppose so . . .'

'Where is your family from?'

'I mean, my dad is Jamaican . . .'

At this point it almost felt necessary to check she was familiar with the concept of slavery – as, apparently, she seemed to be working under the assumption that this name had been handed down over generations, rather than branded on some unfortunate ancestor, the mark of the man who 'owned' them.

Hutchinson (or Hutchison) was the surname of several British property owners in Jamaica in the 1700s. This includes Lewis

Hutchinson – whom I can only *hope* I am not directly related to, given that as well as being a slave owner, with all the brutality that entailed, he elected to throw a little serial killing into the mix.

According to the limited online sources available, he would lure unsuspecting travellers onto his land, only to shoot them, disposing of their bodies in a sink hole, affectionately termed 'Hutchinson's Hole'.

One thing that could be said of him, was that at least he was an equal opportunities offender – he may have kept black slaves, but the victims of his extra-curricular activities seemed to all be white. This no doubt considerably increased the likelihood of him being punished, and he was duly caught and hanged.

Regardless of history, having this surname, apparently reverberating with echoes of tea, crumpets and cricket played with a straight bat, has no doubt at some point provided some benefits. It is well documented, demonstrated in multiple studies, that job applicants with non-European-sounding names face discrimination in the job application process. They are less likely to be called for interview, and even when they are, the panel will no doubt have formed prejudices before they walk through the door.

Even within medicine, despite the automatic points-based shortlisting for specialty training schemes, once you're called into the interview room, the gloves are off. In the time between the panel picking up your CV from the pile and you crossing the threshold, they will have had ample time to start constructing your persona in their mind. All of this no doubt contributes to the aforementioned gap in 'appointability'.

Patients will also be influenced by a doctor's surname. There has been less research on this, but in one US study, patients were surveyed using identical physician profiles, randomly allocated a stereotypically white, African American or Middle Eastern name. Setting aside the potential for career-ending levels of racist faux pas in deciding which 'black names' to include when designing such a study, patients showed a preference for the 'white-sounding' doctors, and were more likely to choose to see them. In the US, this has a direct impact on a doctor's success – in a private healthcare marketplace, being popular is good for business. To thrive, you're just as well learning branding and social media marketing as you are Anatomy and Pharmacology.

Although we may not like to talk about it, (whisper) some doctors in the UK do private work, often the most well-off, Jaguar-driving, golf-loving among us. The patients who can afford this will shop for healthcare like they do everything else. Alongside not-so-subtle signals of alma mater (MA, Oxon, Cantab), lists of prestigious training positions and awards in the biography on the private clinic's website, the right surname inspires confidence. Even within the NHS, it's not hard to see how this sort of preference could bleed into other areas of the doctor–patient interaction – from responses to satisfaction surveys, to the likelihood of receiving complaints.

Of course, this sort of prejudice travels in both directions. Healthcare staff are host to the same unconscious biases as everyone else. Reading a non-European name on the notes of the patient we are about to call, we are liable to make all sorts of assumptions, ranging from their likely comprehension of what we'll say, to the medical and lifestyle factors affecting their health.

At the time, I couldn't fathom if she was trying to make a point, or was just genuinely thick when it came to the subject of history and my name. A more charitable interpretation would simply be well-meaning interest and enthusiasm, unfortunately shackled to a blundering lack of sensitivity. I fear this would be letting her off too easily, however.

Sticking to my script, I resumed the front-of-house-at-the-Ritz (hair policy allowing) routine, asking her if she needed any help with her things on the way out.

* * *

At the end of the clinic, I sat down for a debrief with Imogen, the consultant whose name would be appearing at the top of the clinic letters I sent out. This isn't guaranteed; some less interested consultants are happy to just leave you to get on with it – consigning certain patients to see the SpR at every visit, and wouldn't care if said customer couldn't pick them out of a police lineup.

She was a bit of an enigma; she clearly cared about the patients and the medicine, but there was also the suggestion she didn't *need* the job – every now and then alluding to familial ties to what sounded like unspecified European aristocracy. She was a relatively new consultant, the years of being an SpR not so far behind her that she had gone over to the dark side – as happens to some, who retain minimal interest in teaching and in mentoring.

As well as supervising me clinically, she was my educational supervisor for the year, charged with making sure I was actually learning something on the job.

'See anyone interesting?'

The word 'interesting' could be taken several ways. The model answer would be that they were all interesting, and that their human stories gave me valuable insights into medicine and the human condition. But I was sure in this case she meant anyone presenting with florid or unusual symptoms – limbs about to drop off and the like.

'Not really . . . not besides the people we already discussed.'

In reality, I was still at the stage in my training where if anything even remotely challenging came up, I was expected to come and let her know mid-clinic – hovering outside her door like a child outside the headmaster's office until she was free.

'Margaret Worthing is a bit of a *character*.'

'Oh yes, she *is* miserable. Sorry, I should have seen her myself. How was she?'

I decided not to go into the full detail.

'As you say, miserable . . . although that might be because we don't ever really do much for her.'

'Yes, that's probably right – but better than blowing her up like a balloon with steroids for a disease she doesn't have.'

This is undoubtedly true. There are patients without a hint of provable inflammatory disease who, through a combination of persistence and their consultant's desperation to do *something*, have ended up labelled, and then treated with immune-suppressing treatments.

'Learning how *not* to do things to these patients is an important part of the job. You really need to learn all of the routine rheumatology stuff in the first year – it gives you time to focus on the actually cool stuff.'

In the first year? She had high standards and a habit of just assuming I could live up to them. And she was also a force of nature. Despite her diminutive stature, even in rooms filled with the most cut-throat, 'big deal' consultants, she had perfected the art of speaking without drawing breath to avoid interruption. She often sounded like an auctioneer – pummelling any dissenters into submission with a barrage of salient points and good sense.

'Now, have a look at this scan . . .'

She tended to attract tertiary referrals for the weird and the wonderful, gaining a reputation for sorting out the undiagnosable when they stumped others, at an unusually early stage in her career.

On the screen, the outline of a human form was visible, cut cross-sectionally like a Damien Hirst sheep. Amid the swirling grey of bone and organs that appeared and dissolved as she scrolled through the scan, there were brilliant solar flare hotspots highlighting the location of inflammation, and the cause of the patient's misery.

CHAPTER 7

'Heducation'

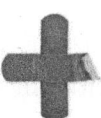

I WAS THE medical SpR in A&E, among the least envied jobs in the hospital, suddenly expected to both treat the person in front of you and supervise junior colleagues, with eyes apparently capable of swivelling in all directions simultaneously, like disco lights.

I had managed to steal a few minutes to actually see my own patient. He came in swaying onto the acute take – if he weren't otherwise immaculately turned out, you'd jump to the conclusion that brandy, or Wray & Nephew were to blame (the drinks choice of many an adult in my family over the age of 50 at parties growing up). Short grey afro hair poked from underneath a brown pork pie hat, and he wore a paisley tie I imagine he had kept pristine since 1960.

He couldn't put one foot in front of the other, and examining his eye movements, for a change there was actually something to see – on this occasion the test wasn't a performative box-tick to satisfy the post-take consultant. As I asked him to follow my finger, they skipped one way and then drifted back to the centre involuntarily, a sign known as nystagmus.

'It just come on all of a sudden.'

He had the same gentle Jamaican accent as my grandparents, the type that soothes as you hear it, coating the air like molasses.

'Okay, and is there anything that makes it better?'

He chuckled. 'Lying down and doing nothing.'

His wife looked at him in a way that suggested this would not be an acceptable new status quo. She was equally church-ready, the visual ideal of the generation who came to the UK in the 1950s and 60s.

Dizziness is up there with headaches when it comes to irritating symptoms when it presents acutely (I mean this selfishly, for me). In almost everyone it will be something innocuous, if unpleasant, like viral labyrinthitis, but a minority will catch you out. Without wanting to spark a wave of hypochondria and flood ED departments, a stroke at the back of the brain can have many of the same symptoms. Admittedly, they tend to be far more dramatic, and are associated with other features that make the diagnosis clear, but not always.

This is another presentation that calls for those seemingly bizarre tests of coordination. 'Okay, now take your right index finger, and touch your nose – then take the same finger and touch my finger. Then go back and forward between my finger and your nose'. Even explaining this specifically, and very *slowly*, patients inevitably don't understand what you're asking, looking like they're attempting a secret Masonic handshake with their face. The assessment can be so difficult that a few strange and dedicated neurologists devote their careers to investigating and treating dizziness.

'Okay, it's probably a problem in your ears.'

'He's deaf alright, when it suit him.'

'Yes, well, in this case, there's a part of your ear that helps you balance – and if you catch a virus, it can stop working properly.'

'It going to get better?'

'Yes, if it's just that, it should. But I'm sorry, you'll have to come into hospital tonight. We need to do a few more tests to make sure it's not anything else – including a stroke.'

This was followed by another familiar sound. He kissed his teeth. 'A stroke . . .'

'It probably isn't,' I assured them, rowing back slightly, 'but it's just better to be on the safe side.'

His wife unleashed a similar but distinct look, another in a repertoire honed over 50 years of marriage, which said, 'you'd *better* do what the doctor says now'.

And, like that, he migrated onto the 'seen' side of the list – shuttled off to the ward to wait for an MRI, a timeframe which, thanks to lack of investment in radiology, is often measured in days.

The surprise would come a couple of months later, when, via my dad, I heard the man I had treated knew my uncle Alf – my dad's eldest brother. In many ways, they couldn't be more different. Like me, my dad is around 5ft 7, but has been rocking the same clean-cut, normcore style since I can remember.

Alf, on the other hand, is over 6 feet tall (a colossus by our family's standards), and a rasta. Whereas my dad sounds like Geoffrey from *The Fresh Prince*, Alf's accent remains Jamaican to the point of defiance – despite having lived over here, in Birmingham no less, since he was 19.

As kids, going over to his house was like stepping into another world. The back room was filled with wicker furniture and pan-African artefacts, and the analogue warmth and crackle of roots reggae vinyl records.

For all his rebellion and contempt for the Babylonian structures of authority, there is, however, very little he holds in higher esteem than knowledge and educational attainment, medicine in particular. His pride at my brother and I being doctors is so complete, that bragging gives way to exaggeration. When I was an FY1, half of Birmingham were almost certainly being told I was a world-famous neurosurgeon pioneering the first head transplant.

He enthused that his friend had been impressed by my bedside manner. I didn't have the heart to remind Alf that I had ended up committing a man to the hospital for what *did* turn out to be a simple case of labyrinthitis.

My uncle's reverence for medicine and all scholastic achievements is, in no small part, down to the environment in which he and my father spent much of their childhoods in Jamaica.

* * *

My only memories of the place are those of a ten-year-old, much of their substance the impressionist collage of a child's mind, and we no longer have any close family members in Jamaica to confirm what has changed. In the far north-east of the island, in Portland, among the more tranquil of Jamaica's parishes, the imaginatively named Long Road creeps along the coast. Hamlet-like clusters of houses bud from the highway's main trunk.

The one time we visited as a family for three weeks in the late 1990s, although calm, it was rural, rugged. Local kids walked barefoot across stones and through what was, to our London eyes, the wild and knotted jungle behind the beach. They could throw rocks in a way that made my brother and I seem like lank-limbed toddlers by comparison – knocking down mangoes and almonds with a force and precision I could never match, even if given a lifetime of practice and a generous dose of steroids.

It had been my first time on a plane – the excitement of the in-flight age-inappropriate film (*Primal Fear* if you're curious) only matched by what, in retrospect, was the most dramatic landing I will hopefully ever experience. Buffeted by the currents coming off the mist-cloaked blue mountains on the approach, we hit the runway hard and bounced, with enough force to unhouse the oxygen masks from overhead. My brother and I were oblivious to any danger; if anything it just enhanced the whole experience. The same couldn't be said of my mother. A nervous flyer at the best of times, this was almost enough to swear her off air travel for good.

I spent the first few days dazed by the heat, humidity and language I didn't recognise as English. There were people who spoke with Jamaican accents back home, but how our new friends greeted us was on another level entirely. It was hard to tell where one word finished and the next began – and many of them I'd never heard before anyway.

When kids asked, 'You 'ave five dollar fi bag juice?', I had no idea they wanted to know if we had enough money for the polythene sacks of radioactive-coloured frozen ice that were everywhere. They were stacked high in freezers in the small kiosk shops, places so full the owner looked wedged in behind the counter by enormous tin drums of processed cheese and bags of homemade coconut drops.

As we gradually grew accustomed, many locals revealed a deep knowledge of the identity of local flora, insects and fish, blended with some slightly folksier wisdom regarding what to do if you were stung by them. I was petrified of stepping on coral, or being bitten by a spider or 'forty legs', the cartoonishly gruesome-looking centipedes.

'That one, if it bite you, give you a stone bruise.' Not wanting to appear clueless, I nodded along.

The family trip home for my dad was not a luxury holiday. This was not resort Jamaica – no curly straws and umbrellas in the coconuts, no throng of tourists with questionable intentions cruising Montego Bay. Alf and my two cousins Liam and Heli were already being put up in what space there was at his aunt Pearl's home. We would be staying with a distant friend, someone my dad had never actually met. The four of us shared the spare room – my brother and I on a spring-loaded fold-out cot on the floor.

Ms Richards was a woman who in my mind could be anywhere from her mid-forties to late fifties, such is the fluid and wildly inaccurate age-estimating ability of a child. She had a short-cropped, squared-off afro, salted white, and lived with her two teenage sons. The older of the two, Troy, pounced almost immediately on the Walkman we had brought over with us, and invariably could be heard warbling tunelessly to Michael Jackson.

'Troy, can I have it back now please?'

This would go ignored as, eyes closed, he kicked and shuffled on the veranda in his string vest in time to the music that was only audible to him.

She was well-off by the standards of the area, with relatives in America sending money and luxuries back home – a satellite dish jutted out from the side of her home like the figurehead on a ship. The intense sense memory lingers of numbingly sweet iced tea, and cornflakes with the equally sugared, caramel taste of condensed milk at her breakfast table.

Long Road was in a state of disrepair apparently stereotypical of the island. Deep, wide potholes scarred the tarmac, and in places driving required such creative navigation as to render the road markings useless – entrusting a higher power to keep oncoming traffic at bay long enough for you to leap back into the relative safety of your own lane.

The road also gave us an insight into the machinery of local corruption, the oil that greased the gears. During the visit,

Dad found himself speaking with a minor politician, sitting at a lunch table set up outside of the small hut his uncle, Mr Douglas, kept on a local beach. The visitor was light-skinned, as is so often the case within the Jamaican socio-economic hierarchy, looking almost Mediterranean. He wore a white linen shirt, sleazily unbuttoned to just above his navel. Tortoiseshell sunglasses on his head nestled in his slick curls.

Even at a young age, the level of deference shown to this man seemed odd, but now I understand, that's just how things get done – not only there, but anywhere a person might want a planning application to go their way, or to open a business. He understood this, and pressed his advantage, the peak moment being him holding aloft a scotch bonnet pepper and exclaiming: 'These, they're just not hot enough.'

Anyone who knows, knows – complaining that even the mildest of scotch bonnets isn't hot enough is like complaining your glass of water isn't wet enough. Nevertheless, there were murmurs of agreement from Mr Douglas. Point seemingly made, he returned to his topic.

'We have colleges here you know! You ever think of coming back?'

Much of his focus seemed to be finding out what it would take to lure my dad to return to Jamaica – lending the prestige of a biochemist plucked from one of Britain's great scientific universities to whatever vaporous project he was dreaming up.

Dad attempted to deflect the question. 'Well, we're very settled in London . . .'

He made the mistake, however, of letting slip something the guy thought he could use to his advantage: 'It does feel like you're taking your life in your hands going anywhere by road here.'

Not 48 hours later, we awoke to find a stretch of road

250 metres long, between Ms Richards's house, where we were staying, and Aunt Pearl's, was being newly tarmacked – and would soon be suitable for even the most timid of British drivers.

Our guide, and in many ways fixer while we were there, was my dad's childhood friend. 'Brown shoe', or just 'Brown', was so called, imaginatively, because of a pair of shoes he had worn to school on the first day. One item of clothing, and it was enough to brand him for life. I couldn't tell you what his job was exactly – handyman, doer of all things – but there wasn't a person he didn't know in the community.

Brown arranged everything while we were there – introducing us to friends, taking us to hidden beaches. On one occasion, Mr Douglas took us out on his fishing boat. A little rougher than a pleasure cruise, the fibreglass hull left microscopic splinters that stung for the rest of the day, and there wasn't a lifejacket in sight. My mother gripped my seven-year-old brother so tightly it drained the little pigment there was from her fingers. It was made worth it, however, when Brown cooked the catch back on the shore over coals in the sand – in a scene worthy of the most engineered and idealised of travel doc food vignettes.

The rural night life was provided by bars often rudimentally assembled from breezeblocks and a counter. The measures were free-poured, strong enough to catch the uninitiated by surprise. The local is the same the world over, in that there will always be some patrons who don't know when to go home, day after day. Here they stood debating loudly and propped unsteadily against the tables in the front yard.

I can remember, on hearing my dad was a doctor, a man with bloodshot and yellow-tinged eyes was presented to him. Dad struggled to explain that he wasn't *that* type of doctor, and having a PhD didn't qualify him to dispense medical advice.

'What can you do for him?'

Staring at the swaying figure in front of him helplessly, Dad went for the safe, blindingly obvious option.

'He needs to drink more water.'

One particular bar was the final stop off on the way home. My parents would buy tiny bottles of rum cream (Bailey's tropical cousin), drinking them as we walked along the dirt track that led up to the house – soundtracked by the crickets coming to life in the brush, the fading light giving way to the bobbing glow of fireflies.

The holiday was capped by a trip from Portland to my grandfather's house in Spanish Town, cutting into the centre of the island in a convoy of two faltering hire cars. The older, more worn vehicle was a white Lada, which needed a push-start more than once, and carried the ever-present risk of breaking down completely, stranding us left to the mercy of the highway.

Luckily, we were driven by dad's cousin Vernal. He was a tall, wire-framed man, with thick square glasses that now wouldn't seem out of place perched on the nose of a Hackney graphic designer, but at the time looked as if they were government issue. Despite being another member of our family who had suffered a lifetime of poor health from sickle cell, he ran a successful island-wide trucking business, so knew the roads intimately and shepherded us there safely.

The house was built to be the conclusion, the crowning glory of my grandfather's migration story – the triumphant return home. Everything was new, the kitchen arrayed in the finest 1990s appliances and Formica. It was single-storey, but the ceilings were so high, the recessed spotlights could only be changed with towering ladders.

His dream was that this would be the new focal point for the family, with younger members making the pilgrimage back to reconnect with our roots. The sticking point was that no one wants to go on holiday to Spanish Town. The place is a land-locked suburb of Kingston that, when the temperature rises, crackles in the still heat. There is little to do, and there is the ever-progressing creep of violence from the capital. The house stood as a white elephant, empty much of the time, a monument to the truth that you can never really go home again.

When my grandfather died in 2019, the biography in the order of service contained a final surprise – not a secret, just a detail that had never come up. Namely that before becoming a baker, growing up in Jamaica, for a time he had lived on a farm, and had worked the land during his childhood and the early years of his adult life. This brought the allotment he maintained in Birmingham, but none of us ever visited, into new perspective.

* * *

My father had lived around Long Road from the age of three – his parents suddenly replaced by his Aunt Pearl, his mother's sister, as they departed Jamaica for 'the Mother Country', seeking the opportunity of a better life. They promised to send for him as soon as they were established, a window that remained open for some 13 years before he was able to finally join them.

Pearl was the area's chief nurse – a role that, alongside stitching the local population back to together, required her to be part public health officer, part administrator, part citizen's advice bureau. She worked out of a low-rise concrete health centre with a corrugated roof, where people would bring their sick child with a fever, or their foolhardy brother whose hunger and gastronomic curiosity had gotten the better of them, and rewarded them with barracuda poisoning.

Pearl was married to Mr Douglas, and he towered over the

house. He was a police officer who had worked all over, at the time when guns seemed to flood the streets of Kingston overnight. Big in every sense, between his revolver and his stories of showdowns and shootouts, it was like living with the black John Wayne. In my mind, wherever he walked, the song 'Bad Boys' from the TV show *Cops* echoed.

His surrogate parents were the very definition of small-town respectability – Ms Pearl walking down the street was accompanied by a rippling wave of removed hats and reverent greetings. This was a time when cursing, or any other misbehaviour around any 'big people', not just your parents, could reward you with a fully sanctioned beating. Even the baddest kids were on their best behaviour.

The supreme importance of everything 'proper' permeated everywhere – including the home. Church on Sundays and prayers at bedtime were a given. One night when a hurricane was bearing down on the community, a friend had come to take them to shelter somewhere safer. As he went to usher Dad and Alf out of their shared room, he was dismayed as they remained kneeling at the edge of their beds – because they hadn't finished that evening's appeal to the lord. Clearly the wrath of God, as visited by Aunt Pearl, conjured more dread than the eye of a tropical storm.

'Gentle Jesus, meek and mild' was quickly interrupted by a hoiking at the scruff of the neck by their rescuer, snapping them back to reality and their current predicament.

This discipline and expectation extended to school, where grades and behaviour were valued above all else. This, coupled with the fact my father was, in his own words, 'a sickly child' when he was very young (so slight he was nicknamed 'spider'), meant that the classroom was the place he had the strongest chance of being the best.

It's oversimplistic to say that this environment is the reason he ended up in his job, but seeing the respect afforded to healthcare workers, able to bend an understanding of biology to the purpose of helping others, left its mark. Or perhaps he was just good at science in school. It would be stupid (and a lie) to argue that having two biochemists as parents didn't then influence my brother and me, both of us going into medicine. It's as if Aunt Pearl found a way to rewrite the genetic code of our family, through force of will alone.

My father's childhood was one of alternating privilege and deprivation. For a child, separation from parents, even for their own eventual benefit, is an injury that can last a lifetime, but living at the health centre, he was treated well, a surrogate child. They lived in a modern house on site, and at times there was even a housekeeper also living there.

At eight, he was wrenched from this home by the first money sent back from England – and the supposed elevation of being packed off to boarding school in Kingston. Like many things in Jamaican society, these were colonial reflections of their English counterparts – populated by the scions of the 'great and the good'. Alongside the three Rs of reading, writing and 'rithmetic, the school specialised in the three Ds of discipline, discipline and discipline.

Senior school forced yet another move, and he was transplanted to live with a maternal uncle, in a house dominated by his wife. The story of the unwelcome stepchild may be well-worn and often flawed, but from the outset, in comparison to their son, he was a second-class citizen.

Their son could do no wrong – and even when he did, it was almost no doubt under my father's deviant influence. As a man in his seventies, Dad still bears the scar on his forehead, from when his cousin threw a stone and struck him between the eyes. Victim or not, he still found himself in trouble – presumably for leading such a good child astray, and bleeding on the good rug.

Staying there however did allow him to attend another famous traditional bastion of education, which meant that by the time he finally arrived in the gloom of 1960s Birmingham, aged 16, he was in many ways more English than the English. He knew the countries of the Commonwealth, and could recite passages of Shakespeare from memory – all qualities *certain* to endear a child to their classmates in a neighbourhood of factory workers. The saving grace was that this most English education was equally rigorous when it came to sport. As a result, despite his meagre frame, he could play cricket better than anyone (at least if his no doubt *gospel* retelling of the glories of his youth are to believed).

The migration can only have been destabilising – swapping the tropics for the place you would see snow for the first time. Sharing a room with siblings you had never met, and living by the rules of parents who were, in many ways, strangers. The relation-ship will always be complicated, the friction between blood, duty and reality.

Careers counselling in the early 1970s was even more scant than the poor advice I still hear given to youngsters considering science or medicine. He needed time to work out what he wanted to do – black kids were hardly being waved into academia at the time. Gap years come in many forms. After school, Dad didn't head off to Africa or India to find himself, swapping one developing nation for another. Instead, he worked.

Over summers, he had always worked in the bakery with his father and his uncles, with all the early starts and night shifts, and then at a bottle-top factory – which, no way to sugar-coat it, can only have been as interesting as it sounds. After school, he

chanced upon a lab technician position at the Midlands Hospital
for Neurology and Neurosurgery, and for the next three years was
responsible for ensuring that the blood and spinal fluid ended up
on the correct analyser, rather than in the bin. This cemented what
he already knew: he wanted to work in medicine, but without the
complicating factor of actually having to interact with patients,
instead remaining one of the scientific wizards behind the curtain.
And to go far in this line of work, he would need a PhD.

Eventually he was liberated, fleeing south to Queen Elizabeth
College in leafy Kensington (now absorbed into King's). There,
he became acquainted with the finer points of biochemistry, and,
more importantly, met my mother. This was at a time when
simply going out in public in some places, especially as a mixed
couple, risked being chased by the National Front.

* * *

Kids are terrible accomplices. They'll always snitch on you
– nothing is in confidence. You gave them ice cream and let
them watch TV all morning to subdue them, securing a rare,
precious moment of peace? Your partner, the one with whom
you agreed to a programme of outdoor activities and educational
nurturing, is going to find out. Away from home, they will repeat
anything you tell them, transmitting to the world – with an
unconscious preference for the profanity and opinions you'd rather
remained private.

'My mum says whites go for whites, and blacks go for blacks.'

Shocking as it might have sounded, delivered by an innocent
freckle-faced child through the gaps in her teeth, in repetition this
was stripped of much of its malice. It was simply something little
Lucy had heard at home, but not fully understood.

'Oh, does she? That's interesting . . .'

This was the sound of Mum's suspicion being confirmed – that Lucy's mother's beliefs matched the Millwall kits the kids received every Christmas. (To be clear, I have friends, or at least friendly acquaintances, who support Millwall, but that doesn't change the overall vibe.) Becoming hyper-alert to racism is a novelty that arrives in adulthood for the white parents of black children.

'Well, that *obviously* can't always be true.'

Her meaning, and the accompanying nod in my direction, must have been all but lost on Lucy, but she felt it needed saying nonetheless.

In what is no doubt a heavily remixed memory, the two of us were sitting on tiny orange, plastic primary school chairs, while my mum sat on a large green beanbag. She was in school that day, as she was among the parents with the time and inclination to come in on a free morning and help kids with reading. While this is admirably community-spirited, even at that young age, having her come into school wasn't exactly the shot in the arm I wanted for my reputation. It's never good to provide people specificity when composing the 'your mum' jokes that form the bedrock of playground insults.

Like my dad, she had trained as a biochemist and received a PhD. The reality of two kids on two salaries reliant on precarious grant funding was a financial and mental strain. She worked part-time in academia for a while, but ultimately traded one lab for another – ending up teaching science to the often-disinterested youth of south-east London.

By now, she was used to fielding the wide-ranging opinions on inter-racial families that could seemingly be unleashed at any moment, by anyone. These could range from the 'oh adorable . . . I think, one day, we'll all look like you' to the 'it's not natural, stick to your own' variety. Although more often offered up by white strangers, this could come from elsewhere. The Nation of Islam, with their well-documented opinions on mixing, were often visible, and I can remember their stern looks as they handed out 'educational material' at the community festival People's Day in Lewisham.

Her father had been an engineer in the navy, running the engines on a destroyer in the Atlantic during the Second World War. The furnace bowels of a ship that might at any point attract the attentions of a U-boat torpedo sound hellish, but being in the navy did mean he'd travelled and worked alongside a more diverse range of people than he might otherwise have done staying in Chatham. When my dad arrived on the scene, he greeted him more warmly than was the norm for the time (even if this shouldn't *really* be the acceptable benchmark).

Likewise, her mother, originally from Glasgow, and who retained the city's lack of pretention, and eschewed English airs and graces (despite apparently having worked in service briefly at the end of the *Downton Abbey* era), met my dad as she would any other potential son-in-law. The same couldn't be said for Mum's uncle – who, on finding out about the relationship, said things I have never heard repeated, so will have to use my imagination (always anxiety-inducing, in case you overshoot, go too big, too racist).

He may have overplayed his hand slightly, since it's not often that vague fondness for an uncle you see occasionally trumps your university boyfriend. The added sting he didn't count on was that my grandmother, his sister, would never speak to him again.

White parents of mixed children find themselves in an odd situation – a sudden radically changed relationship with, and need for awareness of, racism. It doesn't need pointing out that of course they have enjoyed the luxury of years basking in blissful ignorance. There are suddenly places and people they need to be wary of – what does that tattoo say? Is that skinhead a statement or just genetics (or both – anger at male pattern baldness fuelling racial hatred)?

The murder of Stephen Lawrence cast a long shadow over the 1990s in south-east London – the bleak suburbia of Eltham that incubated his killers was a short bus ride away from Catford. And some pockets of Lewisham didn't feel much different. As we got older, would she need to worry about the same thing happening to us?

That morning in school, Lucy, who lived in one of these England flag, pub-strewn enclaves, struggled and battled her way through the rest of the book valiantly, and Biff and Chip overcame their travails. As the lesson drew to a close, my mum couldn't help a parting, 'Tell your mum I say hi.'

* * *

It is just over 75 years since the *Empire Windrush* docked in Tilbury, Essex. This marked the start of a period of migration, during which migrants from Britain's Caribbean colonies settled in the UK. Under the British Nationality act of 1948, they were granted British citizenship, and came after enticement by the UK industries seeking workers to rebuild after the Second World War.

Many went to work in public services, including in the NHS. It is not an exaggeration to say that in the early years after its formation, the health service would have been unable to expand and function without the imported labour of nurses and other professions from the colonies.

Despite being called over to pick up the slack, the welcome often didn't match the initial overtures. Looking for housing, black families were denied, and the infamous 'no Blacks, no dogs, no Irish' signs are not a myth. At work, often things were no better, with some patients refusing to be seen by Caribbean staff. One nurse, Margaret Hazel, speaking to ITV News years later, recalled being told: 'Don't put your black hands on me!'

It takes a real dedication to bigotry to take time out of dying to remember to be racist.

My grandmother had worked as a teacher in Jamaica, but on arriving in the UK, despite the fanatical dedication of the system to the curriculum of the mother country, she found her credentials were unrecognised. Not discouraged, she repeated her training, and was still tutoring local West Bromwich kids well into her seventies.

Still with us, she is a biological marvel. Apparently a born globetrotter, she now lives in North Carolina, but at 96, she recently jumped on a plane and came back to Birmingham, without being morbid, knowing it might be the last time she was able to. My dad and I dutifully took my daughter, who was one at the time, up on the train, so Nan could meet the latest of her now many great-grandchildren.

As we pulled up to the house, her tiny 5ft 4 figure peered excitedly through the net curtains, and then disappeared as she bounced out to greet us.

'Where's my great granddaughter!?'

More agile and animated than many people half her age, the pictures of her holding my daughter are among the most cherished I have. The next generation in the embrace of her roots, the older grasping confirmation that the next was doing just fine.

CHAPTER 8

Where My Mind Is At

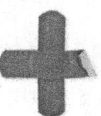

COMING TO THE end of my time in the safety of the gleaming academic Magisterium, I was rotating away from the centre, back to the outer reaches, back to the Trench. This time however as a registrar, facing the prospect of not just having to swim in the chaos, but instead marshal the tides.

I'll be careful, very clear to make the distinction that this is not a bad hospital – if it were, I'd tell you. Because they do exist, and I'd happily risk burning my bridges with any of those places in the hope it would further reduce my chances of ever having to work in them. The kind of hospitals any doctor worried about a sick parent would drive past, to the place several miles down the road, risking the extra time in the car to avoid being left at the mercy of the unchecked slide in standards in their A&Es and wards.

How do hospitals get so bad? The problems are easier to see when considering failing district general hospitals (bad tertiary centres also exist, but their issues can remain masked by reputation).

A dark synergy between lack of funding, serving large areas with ailing populations and an inability to attract and retain talent among their permanent staff – both clinical and managerial.

No, the Trench isn't one of these: it is home to some of the best doctors I have worked with – experts in their specialty, makers of as sound diagnoses and decisions as you'll find. It's just busy, *extremely* busy – Black-Friday-opening-time busy. To labour the aquatic metaphor, being the medical SpR, trying to manage the flow into the hospital, feels like surfing a static wave, a malevolent hand gradually turning up the intensity, willing you to wipe out.

It's the place you earn the stories with which, as a gnarled veteran, you'll bombard wide-eyed recruits, a tear glistening as it trickles from under your eyepatch.

'We saw twenty patients each a night, all critical, without a break . . . One night, my bladder exploded!'

Before I left for this new trial, Imogen handed me a gift – a copy of the *Larousse Gastronomique*, the classic chef's bible. For context, this was a sign she and the rest of the team had *actually* taken the time to get to know something about me (more on inflicting overly complex meals on my long-suffering loved ones later). Working in that department was among the first occasions in medicine I really felt someone higher up cared what happened to me, was guiding me in a direction. One heartening truth I wish more young doctors knew is that, eventually, when you find your home, your specialty, if you're lucky, there will be people there who let you know you belong.

'Be careful at the Trench. No one's going to give you a Nobel Prize if you spend your life in the coroner's court.'

When it came to the rheumatology, thanks to Imogen's mentorship, I now felt like I had half a chance. I knew how to deal with the obvious stuff, investigate the weird, and ask the boss when I didn't know what to do.

The acute and general medicine, on the other hand, brought the step up in intensity I had been promised, but saying I felt ready would have been false bravado. Although nominally doing the same job as at the Magisterium, at the Trench we could be called on to insert large lines into central veins and drain pleural cavities. Expressing anxiety about this is a prompt for older generations to offer some 'back in my day' wisdom.

To them, I'd say firstly, the variation between hospitals as to whose job these procedures are means years can go by without having to do them (or being given the opportunity to practise) – only to then be expected to turn up ready to start prodding. I believe there's a saying about that, something to do with practice making perfect . . . Secondly, back in the day when medical registrars, regardless of their day job, were let loose with the knitting needles, you probably killed and maimed a lot more patients than we're willing to admit.

Approaching the changeover, I felt like an albatross wasn't hanging around my neck, but rather flapping concrete winged strokes in the pit of my stomach. When the rota landed, however, I was gifted a false start, although one that would prolong the agony of suspense. I would be starting my on-calls with nights on the 'cold' hospital site down the road, with no A&E.

This was supposed to be the rest period, down time as payment for the battering taken during the weeks at the acute hospital – a care home for convalescing registrars, but with traffic fumes from the dual carriageway in place of restorative sea air. The wards on this site were all rehabbing hip replacements and strokes, patients unable to go home because of the fraying, candy floss-weak social safety net in place. I even got an SHO – so between us, there was every chance we'd have things wrapped up by midnight and get some sleep.

The evening handover meeting happened in an office above the main hospital entrance corridor, with windows looking out into an unused dead space between blocks. Presumably envisaged as a courtyard, it had been left barren, the only adornment being a suspended netting canopy, decorated by a collection of expired pigeons.

Given the workload, the on-call teams were small skeleton crews – just the two of us and a lone anaesthetist. Alex, the night SHO (the more problematic me would say minion), and his daytime counterpart were in a mini huddle handing over blood tests to look out for.

The main tension that night was waiting for Muriel, the effervescent Guyanese site manager, to inform us whether staff shortages on the main site would mean one of us being put in a cab and sent to do some real work.

Aware of it or not, she drew out the suspense *X Factor* style, the tension at odds with her upbeat delivery, before, finally: 'No staff issues in the acute hospital.'

We collectively let out a sigh of relief while trying not to look too work-shy.

'But . . .'

Oh God, what's the *Columbo* follow-up going to be?

'They're on black alert, so will probably be sending some patients our way.'

Oh, fine. This isn't really news – the hospital is always on some shade of bed alert, the two worst being red and black, but in reality all seeming similarly urgent, with accompanying frantic messages from managers imploring us to 'discharge patients wherever possible' – as if this would be some revelation to us, and up until that point we had been keeping them around just for the company. Apparently in this case, 'black' meant we had 'negative bed capacity' – so even the invented bed spaces that didn't physically exist had been filled, and patients were sitting in ambulances outside A&E, waiting to be unloaded like foreign produce held up in a customs queue.

The first thing was to claim an on-call room, scuttling in, hermit crab-like – leaving enough in the way of personal effects that there could be no doubt in the mind of anyone who came sniffing that it was occupied, even when I was called away. These had been recently refurbished and were clean, but had the atmosphere of the most existential crisis-triggering Travelodge. The windows offered an elevated vantage point onto the pigeon graveyard.

Once we were done on the wards reviewing the one or two patients who had been flagged as potentially misbehaving, before retiring I told Alex to 'call me if you need anything'. The tacit understanding of course being hopefully he shouldn't 'need anything', unless it was life-threateningly urgent.

'I'm sure I'll be fine.' Alex said this with the weary acceptance of a man who knows he'll be bleeped at 2am, because the powers that be have decided now is the time to send a confused 85-year-old across the borough in an ambulance, and they need a warm welcome to check nothing has rattled loose on the ride over.

Unfortunately, a night spent sleeping in a hospital can be just as destabilising as a sleepless one. The eery quiet walking from the ward once the problematic patients have been tucked into bed. The electric hum and creak from the pipes of the on-call room intermittently shaking you alert, out of that liminal place between sleep and wakefulness.

It was almost a relief when my bleep went off.

'Hi, Matt, it's Alex . . .' He sounded sheepish.

'Let me guess, you *need* something?'

'It's a catheter . . . I've tried twice, and it just won't go in.'

'Okay sure, no problem, I'll come down.' I tried to conjure a tone that conveyed helpful approachability, while still subtly suggesting I was doing him a favour (rather than it literally being my job, which it was).

A urinary catheter – a tube that helps get urine that's stuck in the bladder into the outside world (passed up and in exactly along the route you'd think) – may not immediately spring to mind as an emergency. That is until you have either been in need of one yourself, or have treated someone who does. Imagine the sensation of being forced to cross your legs when desperate, but the sweet relief of finding a toilet never comes. Neither patients, nor their kidneys, like it.

When I arrived, Alex was hovering awkwardly at the foot of the patient's bed, a blue sterile field set up on a trolley, and the detritus from the two failed attempts in a bin bag hanging to the side.

The patient, Keith, a grey man in his sixties who had awoken from an operation earlier that day to find his occasional hernia pain replaced by relentless bladder agony, greeted me with a wince.

'Don't worry, we'll sort this out.'

'Please . . . it's unbearable . . . and that felt like he was drilling for oil.'

I had a closer look at the bin bag, at the yellow tubing that drooped sadly over the brim, and was relieved. There are times in medicine when a tiny titbit of knowledge, some small extra experience, makes a world of difference. On this occasion, I was thankful for that four-month urology rotation grappling with the manhood of Essex.

I had seen the boss use an array of tricks to get in otherwise impossible male catheters. The most extreme of these involved pressing on the prostate to adjust the anatomy (again, via the *other* route you are correctly envisaging) – with the visual effect of looking like he was balancing the patient on his finger like a Harlem Globe Trotter spinning a basketball. Fortunately, on this occasion, I didn't think this would be necessary. We were just dealing with the wrong tools for the job.

'I'll be right back.'

Keith didn't look reassured by this. 'Where's he going?'

I headed to the surgical ward storeroom, and was soon back ostentatiously brandishing what I hoped would be the solution. Alongside its more notable uses keeping the tech and cosmetic surgery industries afloat (with a great deal of synergy between the two), silicon catheters, unlike their droopy latex counterparts, are rigid enough that they won't roll up like a curled slipper at the first sign of resistance.

With the combination of this secret weapon, and some firm, but necessary 'manipulation' (yanking), we were rewarded with liquid gold. The expression of relief that flooded Keith's face as the bag filled was, I imagine, the visage of a man as he attains Nirvana, the onset of a blissful tranquillity.

Whenever someone comes to your aid in situations like this, there can be a mix of gratitude and self-reproach at not being able to handle it yourself. Alex leaned more into the gratitude side of things.

'Thanks! Sorry to have to call you.'

'It's fine, sometimes it helps to "straighten the path", but without doing it so much they start to worry you're playing with it.'

* * *

Ever since my first job, night work, with the shift in sleep cycle and lost hours, has always been ruinous to my mental state.

I am naturally an anxious person – although with most things – work tasks, social situations, public speaking – I can get by. The more existential inevitabilities, the more 'teenage philosophy student', on the other hand, are much more of a challenge. It's a fear that seemed to materialise out of nowhere, with no revelatory trigger, but at aged 21, death suddenly seemed to transition from the abstract to a certainty. Life felt like a conveyor belt, but with the additional perpetual threat of being thrown off early if you're not careful. At its worst, the act of getting into a car, placing yourself at the mercy of the driving skills of the same people bumping into you on the pavement feels like too much.

Having a crippling fear of death as a doctor is, to put it mildly, inconvenient. This is particularly the case when doing inpatient hospital jobs, as this is an environment where the subject tends to come up a fair bit. Even if you're doing everything right, the sick and very elderly do have a habit of dying in front of you. The cognitive behavioural approach of rationalising and putting it out of your mind is repeatedly stared down by the glazed visage of the next expiree.

I was on the receiving end of a double hit – night shifts, but with all the time in the world to ponder. At least in jobs when I had been too busy to think, that included not having the time to ruminate on my own inevitable transition to the gurney in front of me. The journey to and from work, on train, tube and bus, was now however a montage of mawkish window-gazing.

During the days, having 'slept' in the hospital, but not rested, I ricocheted around the empty house aimlessly. I had very little to divert this fizzing nervous energy. Of course I spoke to Louise, but there is a limit to how much any of us want to burden a partner – aware of the strain overdoing it can put on a relationship. While I wouldn't go as far as saying we sit having deep and meaningful excavations of the soul, I do at least have friends I can meet and share the same space with when I need them.

I met Tommy in the third year of university, during the interlude, where for an extra year of study, the university doles out an extra degree to medics – the 'intercalated BSc'. At the time, still thinking I wanted to cut people open for a living, I chose the imaginatively named 'surgical sciences' – the skills from which I have rarely been called to unsheathe since.

For many of us, university is one of the final times in life you form real intense friendships. The hours spent near constantly in one another's company, during classes, living together, distilling something fraternal – as likely to spill over into bickering conflict as anything else. Once we even pathetically came to blows, the middle finger of my left hand dislocated as we flailed drunkenly at one another on a Tokyo subway – followed quickly by my snapping it back into place, making up and getting another drink, not wanting to terminally tank the night out.

Loyal and generous, almost as importantly, Tommy knows about good things. Growing up in the restaurant run by his father, he arrived at university with what, by comparison to the snakebite-sodden hordes, was an encyclopaedic knowledge and understanding of food, drink and nightlife. People called him 'Timeout' after the cultural magazine, such was his ability to tell you where you should be going, what you should be drinking. I remain eternally grateful to be able to outsource this part of my brain, to have someone else learn about wine for me (and of course pour it in my general direction).

Tommy had taken advantage of emergency medicine's (his chosen specialty) desperation to hang on to trainees, and negotiated going part-time, despite not having any of the usual excuses of children, or Olympic rowing ambitions. This meant he was reliably available, midweek and middle of the day, when the rest of the world was grinding away.

We met at a place doing (apparently) authentic Japanese breakfasts that, of course, he recommended. Ours is not a relationship given over to frank and honest discussions of our emotions over rice, egg and mackerel, but there is buried emotion – normally conveyed through stereotypical male antagonism.

'Being on nights, somewhere so bleak . . . too much time on my own just thinking.'

'You're complaining about not having anything to do? Have you thought about sucking it up and not being such a pussy?'

This was delivered with a smile that conveyed warmth, not acid – and, as perverse as it may seem, felt like what I needed.

* * *

Soon enough I was back to the relative psychological respite of the ward and clinics – even if it meant there was actual work to do. I still didn't feel completely normal, however, couldn't divert my attention with the myriad other distractions and projects that normally helped block things out.

And, of course, looming was the next block of nights – these were to be the other end of the spectrum. The aforementioned notorious 'too busy to empty your bladder, let alone empty your baggage around a finite existence and your own insignificant place in a vast universe' kind. Of the two extremes, in this scenario, busy is no bad thing, but another circadian shock could have been enough to incapacitate me completely.

Regardless of how much progress we claim to have made, the ability to seek help at work for mental health reasons still isn't equivalent to physical illness or injury. There is a lingering shame, a fear of being perceived as weak.

In medicine, there is a culture of celebrating grit – being able to tough out the most brutal of rotas, of handling the busiest and most understaffed of shifts without complaining. The aforementioned 'when I was in your shoes . . .' spiel from elders, which just makes things worse, the perception the boss feels you should be taking it all in your stride. In this atmosphere, your mood affecting your ability to work is like a soldier turning up on the morning of a battle with an excusal note from their mum.

I was reluctant to do anything – admitting you have a problem risks you being labelled a 'Trainee in Difficulty' – allegedly a process designed to support struggling doctors achieve the necessary competences during their training. There is enough suspicion of the hierarchy, however, that the instinct is to avoid such visibility. This desire will be magnified in staff already concerned about being singled out on the basis of other characteristics such as race, gender or disability.

You may be subject to extra supervision, almost impossible to hide – with the compounding anxiety of the reputational damage this is likely to bring. Nobody wants to be 'that registrar' – the one at whose name consultants and juniors alike groan when they see it on the rota. There is also the chance of your training being extended, prolonging the torture of annual uprooting to new hospitals and night shifts. And memories are long, the world small when it comes to applying for consultant jobs.

Sometimes, a decision is made on your behalf, by your subconscious. It felt like walking on autopilot heading up to the ward from the office, where I had ostensibly spent the morning correcting clinic letters, but, in reality, only working glacially as my insides contracted into a fist.

Dr Sharp, my new educational supervisor for general medicine, a geriatrician in his early forties, originally from Northern Ireland, was 6ft 3, with the physique of a prop forward. When he grasped the hands of the frail elderly patients on his ward, it was like King Kong enveloping Jane in his grip, however gently. Finishing the hours-long round, he had just left the last patient's room. Difficult to read, but fair to the point of obsession, the dynamic between us since starting had been wholly different from Imogen's friendly mentorship, instead teacherly and more distant. I found myself asking him if he had a minute.

'Not exactly . . .'

Looking drained, I could sense his remaining patience was limited. This can't be taken as callous. We were stood in an asymmetric landscape; he could have no idea I was there to discuss that most dreaded subject – feelings.

'Please . . . it's important.'

I gave my most earnest of looks – the type that suggested a patient *might* just be in mortal peril. With a huff, he gave in.

Outside in the corridor, we were in an uncomfortably conspicuous spot by the electronic doors that jerked and swung open aggressively at the regular flow in and out of the ward.

'I . . .'

It became apparent that the words to explain my situation were anything but straightforward to formulate. From the faltering start, it all then came at once.

'I've got a problem with anxiety . . . and it's now to the point I'm worried it's going to interfere with work.'

This was a blindside, and his expression shifted from impatience to confusion – but this was only the midpoint of the progression, as my non-verbal encore ushered him on. As I felt the familiar heaviness threatening to flood and escape my lower lids, he settled on genuine concern (still accented by the agony of awkwardness, inevitable in almost any middle-aged man of his background presented with this situation).

'Okay, I can see this is upsetting you . . . Why don't you head back to the office. We can speak properly in a bit.'

And we did. We agreed it was inevitable that I'd have to see occupational health if I was feeling this bad (although even now, I'm conditioned to need to emphasise I didn't take any time off). There, I saw a kind but firm nurse, who must have been close to retirement and had long ago decided to tell it like it is. She made me promise, no matter how much I resisted, I would seek some kind of help.

* * *

Data regarding the differences in prevalence and severity of mental illness among doctors from ethnic minorities, as compared to the profession as a whole, are limited – to the extent it's almost impossible to draw conclusions. The few studies conducted in the US have failed to find consistent differences and in one case non-white ethnicity was even protective against burnout. It's likely, however, that the same stressors and burdens that boost rates in the wider population will take their toll on doctors.

The black population in the UK experience worse mental health – both in terms of the rates of illness, treatment and outcomes. For example, black people are more likely to experience mental ill health in a given week than their White British counterparts (23 per cent compared to 17 per cent). Black people are four times more likely to be detained or restrained for mental health reasons, and black men experience ten times the rate of psychosis compared to white men. Much like with other specialties, however, they are less likely to seek help, with roughly half the number actively receiving treatment.

Your ethnicity can impact the diagnosis you receive. As a medical student, I remember a well-meaning, but perhaps by modern standards risqué, consultant psychiatrist exclaiming during a teaching session, 'Schizophrenia is a black man's disease', in a tone that wouldn't have seemed out of place in a 19th-century phrenology lecture. I'm almost certain students these days may have been a little hotter on objecting to the delivery of his lesson content to the medical school administration (well-meaning, and in many ways accurate as it was).

He went on to tell us about a local patient of his, who had a telltale sign he was off his meds.

'Whenever Nev was back in his box, we knew he was in trouble.'

The patient in question, every time he was experiencing psychosis, would move into a specific phone box, along with his possessions. He would seal himself inside, sometimes for days at a time – just his eyes visible through the small porthole he left uncovered. I'm curious as to the toilet situation, but almost don't want to know the answer.

Each time, he would need to be coaxed out, sectioned and restarted on the cocktail that kept him if not completely well, then at least out of his street fort.

One of the consultant's main messages, other than to know the quirks of your patients, was that differing ethnicities and social classes will often be diagnosed and treated differently – even when they present with overlapping or even identical symptoms and behaviours.

Delusions and hearing voices – if you're white and middle class, these may be labelled as bipolar. If you're poor and black, it's much more likely to be schizophrenia, not wholly based on any true difference in pathology, but rather influenced by biases and cultural differences. This is not trivial, as the prognosis can be radically different between the two, especially with accurate diagnosis and treatment.

* * *

Such is the concern among doctors around seeking help, however, and yet the need so great, that a bespoke covert service has been set up. The Practitioner Health Programme allows us to self-refer, slinking off in secret, like some psychiatric love rat to speak to someone, without having to go through a GP. The extra layer of patient confidentiality is designed to reassure that nothing unwanted will get back to the powers that be, and so encourage engagement.

This service was a response to above-expected levels of mental health disorders among healthcare professionals, as laid out for example in a report by the society of Occupational Medicine in 2018. I say 'above expected', but it wasn't really. In fact, it feels like a fairly predictable response to sleep deprivation, overwork and the social isolation caused by weekends, nights and the odd forced relocation to the other side of the country, away from friends and family.

Being able to see someone easily is clearly not the norm. Waiting times for the physical illnesses, which the government actually have a half-arsed go at funding, extend into the far distance. For psychology, you may as well put your name down now, even if you're leaping out of bed and skipping to work every morning, just in case you need help in two years' time. In my case, however, I benefited from what could almost be considered a perk of working in the NHS, if it weren't necessitated by such negative history.

Doctors are not immune to the medical cliches that afflict patients. By the time of my first video appointment with the psychologist (a means of communication that felt novel at the time, but now seems oddly prescient), I was essentially fine – a few weeks of living in the daylight had done the job. I almost felt like sleep-depriving myself, reading some Sartre and listening to the Smiths, just to reconjure some authentic symptoms.

He was young, upbeat and distractingly photogenic – looking as prepped for Instagram as he was a consultation. You could just imagine him: 'Hi guys, these are my top five tips for dealing with that pesky existential dread.'

He went through the standard CBT moves.

'Tell me what you're worried about . . . try and focus on how unlikely that is to happen today, or any time soon.'

Even if this can be effective, it does feel a little like ignoring a hole in your roof because the sun is shining, confidently announcing 'that's future me's problem', and throwing a garden party. But, for now, it worked. I was no longer feeling in the depths, and being able to arrange another appointment when I needed it was valuable. This felt like a life jacket going into the next churning swell of on-calls.

CHAPTER 9

Risky Business

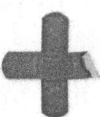

ON THE MEDICAL take, mid-afternoon is when the lunch rush starts. The A&E doctors have referred their morning patients, and those sent in by their GP arrive. They are racked up like kitchen tickets – 1 pneumonia medium severe, 2 NSTEMIs (a type of heart attack) and a diabetic ketoacidosis, extra sweet . . . The central desk may as well be the pass, with doctors de partie and commis bringing their cooked (or so they think) patients for inspection.

'This one needs a bit more fluid . . . and do another gas.'

The SHO diligently disappears to add these finishing touches – although aware this will slow them down, and might dent their numbers for the day, risking the raised eyebrow of the post-take consultant.

The front-of-house nursing staff also have their say, bringing the gripes of customers when they've been ignored for too long, or have a complaint about what has been served.

'Mr Jones in 12 has been waiting three hours. He's complaining – and he's going to breach.'

Breaching – a fate so dreaded and fretted over, you would be forgiven for assuming these patients burst in to flames, incinerating staff and neighbouring patients alike. In fact, all it means is they have been in the department for more than 4 hours without being admitted or sent home. Make no mistake – having standards keeping patients moving is important, but the punishments for departments failing to meet them means you have ridiculous conversations, are asked questions you couldn't possibly have an answer for.

'Doctor, is this patient coming in or going home? They're on three hours forty-five.'

'I don't know – they have literally just been referred. No one from medicine has even met them. Would you like me to flip a coin?'

Now, at this point, some keen soul with a fetish for patient flow will chime in that they should be moved to an acute medical unit (AMU) and assessed there. Great when this system works, but I have yet to work in a hospital where there is always an AMU bed free to move people to, and, even then, one that is stocked with all the equipment necessary to assess a patient to the exacting standards of certain post-take consultants.

'Where is the ophthalmoscope, please?'

'In the equipment room – but the bulb is broken, and the trolley has lost a wheel.'

'Ah, the NHS, envy of the world.' I say this, despite many ophthalmologists agreeing that a retinal examination in un-dilated eyes from a medic is next to useless anyway.

The patient is most likely in a four-bedded bay – if it's night, even a half-arsed examination will wake up their neighbours (not that I'd dream of letting standards slip in the name of a good night's sleep). They're probably asleep themselves, likely to be vexed you're rousing them for the same questions and prodding they were subjected to by the A&E SHO.

At the nursing station, a queue is forming – a drawback of sitting somewhere you can be found . . . They surge when I get off the phone and it looks like I'm free to take a referral – the ED doctors clamouring like 80s brokers trying to dump a bad stock. Shreya is the winner, catching my attention first, and starts her sales pitch.

'He's only forty, doesn't smoke, but says it's the worst chest pain he's ever experienced – does he need to come in?'

The list is already groaning, we have negative beds, and I can just imagine the ridicule if I admit this picture of health and he's having anything less than a full set menu coronary.

'What does his ECG look like?'

She hands me a sheet of reassuring squiggles (technical term) – extra reassuring because the computer-generated cheat sheet analysis agrees it's normal for once. More commonly it reads 'non-specific T-wave abnormality' – meaning 'probably fine, but could also be on the cusp of a heart attack that will be catastrophic for both the patient and your career.'

'Looks fine to me – and you said his troponin [the blood test which becomes abnormal during a heart attack] was negative, and it started more than four hours ago?'

'But he says the pain is *really* bad . . .'

As much as I dislike standing up unnecessarily, sometimes five minutes of leg work can save you hours later.

At the cubicle, behind the curtain is a very healthy looking, but very anxious young(ish) man. Rope-like veins curl and contour his skin, his t-shirt fabric having to work extra hard to contain a physique that appears made up of 90 per cent creatine.

I ask him all the autopilot, standard pain history-taking

questions – remembered with one of the thousand mnemonics medics use to counter the effects of tiredness and forgetfulness.

If you're wondering:

S – Site

O – Onset

C – Character

R – Radiation

A – Associated symptoms

T – Timing

E – Exacerbating/alleviating factors

S – Severity

To be fair to Shreya, he does have a dull, aching pain in the middle of the chest that gets worse when he exerts himself.

'Okay. A couple more questions, Marcus. First, have you been exercising recently by any chance?'

'Yeah, I go to the gym. I've been trying to stay fit since my dad had a heart attack a couple of years ago.'

'And have you been working out your *chest* a lot recently?'

At this, realisation creeps across first Marcus, and then, as if by contagion, Shreya's face.

'I *did* bench quite a lot yesterday' – a line of supreme bro confidence, but delivered sheepishly, like a schoolboy who had just smashed a window playing football.

'I think it's safe to say you can go home.'

At this point, you might expect me to climb on my soap box to bemoan time wasters – clogging A&E with non-problems, calling ambulances because they can't change the channel on their TV, or have too much wax in their ears. This might be valid, but the overwhelming feeling in situations like this is of a win – problem solved, a bed saved, and a number on the board with my name next to it, all in a couple of minutes.

Of course, there is always the risk he'll turn out to have an aortic dissection and keel over on the street outside just to spite me. In the coroner's court, the expert witness drawing everyone's attention to the subtle signs on the chest X-ray heralding the imminent relocation of his circulating volume from his arteries into his thorax – clear as day in their eyes, but missed in the heat of the moment.

Being under pressure to send people home is apparently not an excuse for this sort of thing – this is always worth bearing in mind next time that aforementioned frantic text message arrives from the hospital switchboard warning of 'black alert . . . bed shortage . . . avoid admission wherever possible'. We are operating a night-time establishment with an elastic door policy, and when things get busy, it's one in, one out.

Management are always interested then – you might even see them popping down to the department, MBAs who couldn't read an ECG if the trace spelled out 'happy birthday', or 'I'm having a massive heart attack' – shirt sleeves rolled up, concerned faces bursting with questions about 'what can be done to get things moving?'

When something does go wrong, which statistics and/or the will of a spiteful deity make certain it eventually will, this pressure will be reframed, or forgotten. No one owning up to the instruction to cut corners and kick 'em out ASAP. They will be awfully quiet about their levels of influence once something terrible happens.

When this does happen, there are a few things it's worth remembering to help your career survive the process. Make accurate notes, contact your medical defence organisation, and most importantly, if you can, try to avoid being non-white. It really increases your chances of being referred to the GMC, struck off and even prosecuted – and no one wants that.

Many doctors have found this out the hard way. In February 2011, Dr Hadiza Bawa-Garba returned to her first day in acute paediatrics after maternity leave, to a working environment that could generously be described as a faecal cyclone. A gap in the rota meant she would unexpectedly be covering the ED and emergencies alongside her own job – a gift on a par with being handed one of those turds rolled up into a pain au chocolat at the morning meeting.

The on-call consultant, apparently unable to master the complexities of a calendar, had forgotten he was on call that day – and was instead giving a lecture in another city – hopefully not on the importance of patient safety, diary management or trainee supervision.

During the course of a shift that included being the most senior doctor looking after patients spread across four floors of the hospital and A&E, a child with sepsis died due to a cavalcade of systemic failings. These included the aforementioned unsafe staffing and the IT system going down for several hours, preventing access to blood results – akin to blacking out half of the instrument gauges on a pilot's dashboard.

It can never be forgotten that, at the heart of this story, the tragedy is the death of a child. I'm not expecting anything I write to change the opinion of anyone emotionally invested in the case – that's not how this works. Nor can it be ignored that Dr Bawa-Garba made errors – during the cardiac arrest, she mistook him for another patient with a DNACPR order in place, who had been in the same bed earlier that day, and temporarily stopped the ongoing resuscitation. Regardless, this was determined by the coroner not to have contributed to the death.

She had correctly omitted the patient's enalapril medication from the drug chart – as this could cause a dangerous drop in blood pressure. She didn't also write this instruction in the notes, however – and the hospital had a policy of letting parents administer regular medications to children, before it was prescribed, even when they were acutely unwell – which, as far as policies go, seems, in short, stupid.

Doctors hearing the details of the case, and the punishment handed down, were disturbed – not because mistakes hadn't been made by Dr Bawa-Garba, but because they recognise all too well the situation she found herself in. In the maelstrom that has come to be accepted as 'just another day on call', we know that we could – perhaps even inevitably *would* – make similar mistakes.

We'll put up with coming to a workplace where you're asked to do more with less, hoping we still manage to do a decent job. But if this means being criminalised when mistakes inevitably happen, eventually we will just stop.

Comparisons to the airline industry have become cliche in medicine when talking about patient safety, but they remain the most apt. If on the morning of a flight, the pilot doesn't show up, the plane doesn't take off. You don't pat the first officer on the head and say, 'Looks like you're flying solo today, buddy, oh and also, when you get a minute, we'll need you to man the drinks trolley once you get up there – cabin crew issues.'

Dr Bawa-Garba was prosecuted for manslaughter on the basis of forced errors made under extreme stress. It is hard to ignore race in this – she was born in Nigeria and wears a hijab, which despite what some incensed flush-faced pundits might tell you, is still enough to mark you out. Otherwise, why was her treatment so different from that of the consultant? At least she was there that day.

Non-white doctors are significantly more likely to be referred to the GMC and face sanctions. In 2019, a GMC report found the rate was double that of their white counterparts. Although admittedly a rare event, they are also over-represented in the number of manslaughter prosecutions. In 2018, the British Association of Physicians of Indian Origin examined cases over the preceding decade, and found that of the 20 manslaughter prosecutions, 12 were non-white (this is out of proportion to the ethnic makeup of the UK doctor workforce), as were all seven of the successful convictions.

Among these was surgeon Mr David Sellu. He was prosecuted following the death of a patient at a private hospital. Originally admitted for a knee replacement, the patient complained of abdominal pain and a CT scan showed he had a perforated bowel, requiring an emergency operation.

There were delays – first a wait for an operating theatre and then for an anaesthetist, as no emergency rota was in place. These contributed to the outcome – but Mr Sellu was held accountable. Quite how or why I'm not sure. Short of knocking the patient out himself and operating on the ward, it's not clear what he was supposed to do to get an operation done faster.

Convicted, Mr Sellu was sent to Belmarsh Prison, among her (now his) majesty's least salubrious accommodations – in no small part because the hospital he was working in had inadequate systems for dealing with emergencies. This was confirmed in a report they commissioned themselves, but conveniently neglected to pass on to the GMC or the courts. On appeal, Mr Sellu was cleared of any wrongdoing – but not before he had spent eight months inside.

* * *

It's common knowledge that TV medical dramas bend the truth, and often outright lie. Perfectly coiffed heroes with model looks stride purposefully down corridors, CPR raises hopeless cases – wrestling them from Hades's grasp to live on. The most unrealistic scene by far, though, is the tug of war between specialties over care.

'Back off, medicine, this is surgery's patient!' is a sentence that has never been uttered by anyone in a hospital, ever – at least not in the UK. Sure, there are fights – but they are much more along the lines of:

'Based on the number of comorbidities and age, they need to come in under medicine.'

'But he's got appendicitis!'

'New policy – these elderly patients do better under medicine... with surgical input of course.'

'You can't just look after people badly and get rewarded with less work.'

Today's battle is with orthopaedics – a speciality often maligned out of jealousy more than anything else. They actually get to make people better, fixing their hips and knees, sending septuagenarians back to the squash court – and their spaces in the car park tell you everything you need to know about the private work. People will pay a lot for a new joint if it means walking the golf course pain-free.

'So she's got a fever, a CRP of 300, and pain in her right hip – the hip *someone*, one of your bosses, not so long ago replaced . . . pain so bad she can't stand up – and you *don't* think there is a chance she might have septic arthritis?'

'Why would she just suddenly get an infection in her hip?'

'I mean now we're getting philosophical . . .'

I want to add: 'Because the hip is a joint like any other and gets infected when you start messing around with it, because more weird stuff happens the older you get, or maybe one of you forgot to wash your hands before operating! Just take her you work-shy ego in scrubs' (an accusation which could *never* be levelled at me, of course) – but am forced to hold my tongue because of 'manners' and 'professionalism'.

'I think she needs to come in under medicine – investigate all causes of infection. We can come and review her once she's had an ultrasound.'

There is only so long it's worth persevering with this sort of argument. The orthopaedics registrar was a new ST3 (specialty training Year 3), keen to flex the novel muscular authority the position brings. This can be a risky time in a career; the confidence boost is enough to turn some into a walking Dunning–Kruger nightmare, hubris elbowing out any awareness of what they don't know.

While not doing extra work is pretty high on my list of priorities, doing what's best for the patient edges it. Plus, when the other tests come back negative, and the ultrasound inevitably comes back showing a collection of pus ortho needs to deal with, I'll get the chance to gloat – a moment to be savoured, up there with delivering a baby, or saving a life.

'Fine, but we'll be seeing you tomorrow,' I say with a deliberately concocted blend of world-weariness and menace.

In the time I've been with this patient, service has started getting away from us – things are backed up and I've lost track of which SHOs are seeing which patient, and who should be finishing up, ready to pick up another. The nurse in charge adds the names of three GP referrals simultaneously, swelling the unruly list – just as the post-take consultant arrives.

We are, as they keep reminding us, working in a 'busy DGH', a district general hospital – a large, canteen-like operation, dolling hearty fare and turning the tables. We deal in volume, while doing it safely. It's about seeing the patient, working out as best you can what's wrong, ladling out the treatment and moving on.

We don't have time to be doing the extras, wrapping the patient up in a nice bow to present to the consultant when they arrive – as is expected in some of the more esteemed (and quiet) academic centres. There, if the serum rhubarb levels (a mocking term for the niche blood tests some consultants demand) haven't been checked on that patient with a rash, there will be hell to pay. Most DGH consultants recognise the environment, the lay of the land, and will let you off not doing a 15-minute precision neurological examination on everyone.

That the medical community accept this difference has always disturbed me – hospitals shouldn't be classifiable as 'busy' or 'quiet'. Surely it takes a certain number of doctors to treat a certain volume of patients, and hospitals should be provisioned accordingly. I also know that hoping for those in control of budgets to take notice and change things, is naivety on a par with wishing for world peace, or that salad tasted like steak. But it could be done – we know which hospitals fall apart most catastrophically each winter. We know the average numbers attending each place at different times of the year. Matching resources to average patient numbers wouldn't be that hard, if there was willing (and money).

Dr Malik, the consultant, has silently materialised and is scowling at the sprawling list. She does not look best pleased. The faint atmosphere of *Ramsay's Kitchen Nightmares* is already creeping in, the nadir before that week's mid-episode makeover has occurred, Gordon's craggy face scowling as the hapless staff of the doomed restaurant tank another service for the cameras.

'Is there anyone actually ready for me to see?' she asks indignantly, her facial expression pre-empting my meek, muttered response.

'I'm not sure, let me check the list.'

'Come on, you should be on top of this – you've got to get a grip.'

I start to protest; getting dragged into that futile game of hot potato with ortho is the only reason I've momentarily lost track of things. In reality, how a take goes in a place like this can be as much down to fate as it is the SpR's skills in leadership anyway.

That day's complement of SHOs is key – the old school in me might say some are workers, some are shirkers. It's a big department, and there are lots of places to sit ruminating over a patient (or checking Instagram) rather than pulling your finger out, taking the pulse of the situation and getting on with getting shit done. The modern, reformed me, on the other hand, would accept that there is a diverse range of skill sets, personality types and personal circumstances affecting the amount of time and support staff need. Whichever of those you believe, the outcome is the same – see some faces at the start of the shift, you breathe a sigh of relief; others may as well be blank space.

Everyone knows this, but come handover, the news that there are ten waiting, and several of those who have already been seen are falling apart, is met with the same clenched-tooth contempt from incoming colleagues. This is regardless as to whether you were playing with the A-team all day, or babysitting the under-11s – no one cares about that last-minute busload of patients that rushed the door in the last hour.

I scan the list quickly – it's potluck as to who might have someone ready for inspection. My choice made, I head over to one of the nearby cubicles to see whether I have backed a winner. I poke my head in, to check on Aaron, and am greeted with him pressing a hand to his patient's wrist, looking wide-eyed and frantic. She was a woman in her fifties with bronchiectasis, a chronic lung disease, and had come in with life-threatening pneumonia.

Correctly, Aaron realised she would benefit from intra-arterial blood pressure monitoring and decided to insert an arterial line. Unfortunately, coordinating this with the nurse looking after her has clearly hit a snag. The transducer wasn't set up, the line wasn't flushed in time – meaning the whole thing has clotted off and stopped working, and he has had to pull it out. All that poking around the main artery in her wrist with a big needle, followed by the tinkering and then removal, has made her a bit bleedy. He removes his hand to check the situation, a movement that is met instantly by the crimson spurt and spatter sounds of arterial blood hitting his disposable apron.

Hoping that Dr Malik hasn't witnessed this, I look over my shoulder to see her looming in the doorway. From her face, the pot is clearly boiling over. The rhythmic piston-like jet from the wrist drives home her contempt for the both of us, deepening with each pulsation.

CHAPTER 10

A New Dawn, Old Problems

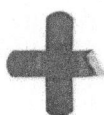

AS A GLOBAL pandemic was inching and then suddenly jumping its way to the UK, you might think, as supposedly highly trained problem-solvers, we would have twigged sooner. One night in early March, I had accepted 13 referrals for suspected pneumonia or breathing difficulty, which even for a bad take was excessive.

Believing the line that it wasn't circulating in the community in the UK, COVID-19 wasn't double-underlined at the top of every differential diagnosis list, as it should have been. And several of them were young; a woman in her thirties with streaks across both lung fields on the X-ray. At this time, protocols for isolation were still being made up on the fly and, for the most part, swabbing was reserved for those travelling from Italy or China. Ostrich-like, we had convinced ourselves it wasn't here yet.

It was only days later, doing my usual remote post-admissions snooping, when I saw that once they had finally been done, the tests all came back with the relentlessly consistent 'positive'. The respiratory ward was soon almost entirely dedicated to COVID, with ambulances dropping off the most red-flag patients straight to a dedicated assessment area.

Writing now, from the comfort of the post-vaccine future, it's almost impossible to reinhabit the mindset from a time when we knew almost nothing – the uncertainty and the fear, how the reassurances from on high felt like an owner telling you their snarling XL Bully is 'perfectly safe'. The first night we knew for definite we may be seeing COVID patients, the advice regarding PPE felt as if someone was freestyling it – matching clinical scenarios and levels of protection by spinning the wheel of misfortune.

'Is CPR aerosol generating?'

(Gameshow audience in unison): 'Fuck knows!'

'What protection do we need when doing it? Let's spin the wheel and find out . . .'

The answer initially (later revised) was that we would be just fine with simple surgical masks. Any sane person considering this for half a second could see it was dumb. As the team member likely to be leading, stood back during a resuscitation, I would be asking the SHOs and others to dive in around the body, sucking in the miasma while they pounded the chest or scoured for veins and arterial blood. I would be responsible, and wasn't going to submit willingly to any 'lions led by donkeys' safety fiasco.

At this time, the medical high-dependency unit (HDU) was still a quaint six beds. They had a stock of FFP3 masks, reserved for the one infectious patient side room, that up until now had been used mainly for cases of flu.

Manny is a kind but vigilant charge nurse. He had been here during my first run through the Trench as an SHO. Highly trained and sharp-eyed, he would stop you from making potentially lethal mistakes – reminding us that if we were prescribing IV insulin for diabetic ketoacidosis, it's usually a good idea to write up enough glucose alongside it, to avoid killing them when the blood sugar inevitably crashes (apparently hypoglycaemic comas correlate poorly with survival).

He's one of the many highly skilled nurses the NHS has "recruited" (stolen) from the Philippines. At times it feels like we have taken half of their workforce. Although there are supposed to be policies in place to prevent 'brain drain' from foreign health systems, and the skill they bring is welcomed, there is still discomfort at the thought of the hole left back home. They should also, of course, be able to move wherever there is a call for their skills, allowed to improve their own lives, as many of our families have done. But there has to be a genuine effort to train and replace more than have been taken.

Rotating back out of clinic land, he was patient with the rust my 'critical care light' abilities had accumulated, this being a hospital with a medical HDU – manned by an often-bewildered parade of non-intensive-care-trained medical SpRs with variable skill sets. Putting in an arterial line after four years away took me what felt like an age of sweat, blood and hand-shaking, but Manny didn't say anything.

Now I had come to him on bended knee. They were sending us into the unknown with little more than a pat on the back and encouraging a stiff upper lip. I explained my fears, namely that we would all be exposed to an infection for which we still didn't have a good grasp of the mortality rate, and our fates would fall under that most sombre category of 'lessons learned'.

'Can I *please* take some of these proper masks? The ones they're giving us look as useful as a string vest in a blizzard.'

He weighed up the request – not unreasonably. The soft PPE guidance was clearly an attempt to ration stocks for what was coming, and anything he gave me wouldn't be available for the HDU nurses later. Then again, in the collegial spirit of the multi-disciplinary team (MDT), whatever we caught out there, we would bring back on to the ward. Sense and kindness prevailed, and I left with what we needed.

* * *

Of course, early on, there were mistakes. Dr Siva, the on-call consultant, had been in and out of the room of a man who was tubed, with a suspected pulmonary embolism. Arriving back from a business trip to Brazil, he had stepped off his flight and promptly collapsed on the runway.

It seemed like a medical school multiple-choice question open goal: funny turn after a long-haul flight? You're a moron if you don't go for clot as the answer. We had been so confident, the CTPA – a scan showing the lungs and their circulation felt like a formality. His blood had been thinned, and we were primed for thrombolysis if he deteriorated.

When the report came back 'bilateral ground glass changes and infiltrates . . . broad differential . . .', the 'consider COVID-19' was almost superfluous and may as well have been followed by 'you idiots'.

Dr Siva looked queasy; his mask discipline had been lax. No one could agree what constituted a high-risk exposure, but at the time, with a tube sitting deep in the patient's airway, this felt one. Since then, a large body of learned, if at times slightly tedious and often contradictory, research from critical care has emerged, defining the sorts of ventilation that blow the most death particles back into the room, what type of tube forms a closed circuit . . . but at the time we were left to guess.

That was him done for the day. He was forced to shower,

change and sheepishly scuttle home to isolate, leaving the second consultant (this hospital having enough admissions to need two) to wade through the remainder of the patients with the take team.

* * *

As the days progressed, more of the hospital was given over to COVID patients, and ITU expanded like some hive organism. Theatre recovery areas and ward bays were sealed off, seemingly sprouting ventilators.

The AMU was also quickly requisitioned. I recall coming in for my first shift on the ward, expecting the usual mix of heart failure, pyelonephritis and blood clots, only to meet the grinning infection consultant freshly commissioning us as the new COVID overflow.

His crystal-blue eyes had upped their intensity, and he stomped around purposefully in his scrubs and white hospital-issue wellies.

The infection and lung doctors seemed to be loving this all a bit too much. Like pigs in shit, it was their time. The lung doctors all suddenly had opinions about respiratory droplet size, work of breathing and lung remodelling during infection. The infection doctors developed acute cases of Cassandra syndrome; this was the pandemic they had been warning of for a long time, though they conveniently forgot that they had been sure it would be flu.

Like firefighters in a Hollywood blockbuster readying to tackle an inferno, they were having their 'this is what we trained for' moment. We forget now, but most people were still calling it 'the Coronavirus'. The first time I heard the respiratory registrar referring to it as 'COVID', the first thought was: *Steady on, who are you trying to impress?*

Before it sounds too much like I'm dumping on everyone else and keeping myself clean, we in rheumatology were not immune from imagining ourselves at the heart of things. It had been noticed early on that many of the patients in the first case series from China looked very inflamed, with similarities in their blood tests to conditions that sometimes fall under our remit. There was a flurry of opinion and review of what scant evidence there was, suggesting we might have the answer (and in the fullness of time, some, but by no means all, of the drugs we use did prove effective).

As things progressed, clinicians observed that the ethnic makeup of the patients coming in was skewed. In our hospital, there was no guarantee we would have noticed. Not because it wasn't happening, or because our workforce was staffed by the type of arch-progressives who 'don't see colour'. Rather, the population we served already aligned with the communities most affected by COVID, so our admissions had looked this way for years.

But it became clear that some were taking the brunt – families where three generations had gradually been admitted over the same week. A middle-aged taxi driver bringing it home from work, infecting his parents, only for his daughter, who had been looking after everyone else, to finally be wheeled in on oxygen.

The pandemic, particularly the early period, had an outsized impact on non-white groups. They were more likely to contract the virus, with members of the Bangladeshi community at an 88 per cent increased risk relative to white counterparts – the worst affected group by this metric. In turn, the same people had a significantly increased risk of being hospitalised and dying.

There are multiple underlying reasons, but key among them are employment and housing. Without wishing to over-stereotype, people in these groups are more likely to work in jobs that make distancing and remote working less easy. You can hardly clean over Zoom. Having contracted the virus, they were then also more likely to take it back to crowded accommodation, where it would then inevitably spread.

Our hospital is renowned as serving this subset of patients, so impacted by diabetes and illnesses of deprivation, that the daily hospital intake has always been a special case unto itself. A higher baseline prevalence of health conditions associated with COVID mortality is likely an important factor in the differences seen. Although it is difficult to unequivocally prove causation, many individuals were almost certainly at increased risk thanks to existing health inequalities.

* * *

When the disparities in mortality due to COVID between ethnic groups were noted, there was a great appetite to find a genetic-smoking gun, rather than focusing on the likely more important social determinants.

For example, a huge amount of time and effort, as well as column inches, was dedicated to the consideration that differences in ACE2 receptors (proteins on the surface of cells that the virus uses to get inside) were responsible. It's not possible to discount a contribution, but based on our understanding of genetic diversity, the likelihood of some single shared gene among all at-risk ethnic groups, who also all happen to come from communities disadvantaged in the UK, is small.

Dual harms loom in research focusing on race. The early 'scientific' establishment demonstrated that it couldn't be trusted. Throughout history, a frankly absurd amount of time was spent by people, including the German philosopher Christoph Meiners, trying to assert ideas related to a racial hierarchy – rankings that would provide justification for colonialism and slavery.

Putting the 'light' in Enlightenment – light in skin, lighter on facts – luminaries of this time including Voltaire had opinions, most of them not too savoury. With very little, or even no exposure to the people they were discussing and classifying, authors opined on their intelligence, supposed lack of a culture, and questioned their humanity.

The idea that race has a true biological basis has been done away with, giving way to an improved understanding of genetics, garrotted by the strands of the double helix. There are no biologically definable races; rather, race is a construct. The science of genomics has demonstrated that, by most metrics, there is greater genetic diversity within individuals on the continent of Africa than between individuals compared across continents.

Racism can cut you twice. There is the initial insult, the injury, followed by the way in which we have to change the world around us, or how we behave, to prevent it from happening again. This will be a dim memory to many now, but in 2018, H&M came under fire for an advert in which a black child was photographed in a hoody emblazoned with the words 'COOLEST MONKEY IN THE JUNGLE'.

To anyone with even the most casual awareness of racial history, this showed about as much sensitivity as a fully anaesthetised Piers Morgan. There were almost certainly no black people with a voice in the room when this was signed off. Associating black people with monkeys and apes is a trope that has long been used to justify treating us as less than. Poster boy for the rights of man Thomas Jefferson (of 'all men are created equal' fame, also owner of 600 enslaved people) made the comparison in 1785, in his 'Notes on the State of Virginia'. Black professional footballers are still taunted with chants and banana skins at matches.

The harm from these acts is obvious. But then the need to insulate against them places burdens and restrictions on black people. Ask a black football fan how likely they would be to follow their team to one of the central or eastern European countries where these chants have recently been heard (or even certain UK grounds, where they also used to be commonplace, for that matter). About as likely as finding Nigel Farage Dutty Wining at Notting Hill Carnival.

In the case of H&M, an innocent child was placed at the centre of a fight they should never have had to worry about – all while participating in an opportunity which, at the time, presumably, had been fun and exciting, but they would no doubt avoid given the chance again. Racism makes us deprive ourselves of things to stay safe and restricts what we can do without fearing consequence.

The same is true in science. The history of science done in bad faith has made it very difficult to research differences in outcomes between ethnic groups, without first having to ensure that what is being done won't be subverted, misappropriated or misinterpreted. Namely that what is being conducted isn't discredited 'race science'.

There is nuance to the relationship between 'race' and genetics. Racialised and ethnic groups with common ancestral links *can* share genes which predispose them to certain diseases. For example, a variant of the APOL1 gene, most common in parts of West and Central Africa, predisposes to certain kidney diseases. It is believed it provides some protection against forms of the parasitic disease African sleeping sickness, explaining the gene's persistence.

External factors such as the transatlantic slave trade can shuffle and concentrate these variants among racialised populations. This APOL1 risk variant is prevalent among African Americans due to the regions on the continent from which their ancestors were taken. During the HIV epidemic, an increased risk of kidney complications (HIV nephropathy) was seen among this group when infected with the virus, due to this mutation.

So, a certain gene or condition *can* become prevalent in a subset of a larger group of people arbitrarily lumped together. But this skews the results for the wider whole. People erroneously arrive at the assumption that a given risk applies to all members of the wider group, for example those considered black. Ascribing this same risk of kidney disease to a recent migrant from elsewhere on the continent, for example from South Africa, where the distribution of the variant is completely different, would make no sense.

And yet this is entirely what many of our current practices do. I wince any time I hear one of my colleagues describe African patients as 'African Caribbean', when neither they, nor their ancestors, have ever travelled further west than Reading. In many instances, kidney and lung function test results are still adjusted for some imagined all-encompassing 'black ethnicity', despite there being no genetic or physiological basis for doing so. The results of these tests are used as the thresholds for intervention in a range of conditions, with the potential to cause delays in treatment, and thus real harm – a point expanded upon in Dr Layal Liverpool's *Systemic*.

As the power of the clinical genetics tools at our disposal increases, and the cost reduces, our assessment of patients will change drastically. Ever since I was at medical school, the era of personalised medicine has been perpetually on the horizon – much like the driverless car, or jetpacks. But, at some point, it will be possible for doctors to obtain detailed information about your genes, and use this to guide treatment. Assumptions based on race, ethnicity or geographic origin will be even more redundant.

When this becomes possible, even more certain than the improvement of health outcomes is the likelihood that information will be misused. It is never wise to underestimate our capacity to create an outgroup.

* * *

'Omar wants to know what his CRP is.'

'He *just* asked fifteen minutes ago – it's not back yet. He's like a toddler in the car.'

Omar had been trying everyone's patience, but only by behaving in exactly the same way we all would in his position. Obsessing over every blood test, every scrap of information that might give some idea what his chances were.

Originally from Somalia, he was one of the career A&E middle-grade doctors that prop up departments the length of the country. He worked in a hospital on the other side of London, but was with us, scrubs swapped for a gown, because he had the misfortune of having caught COVID, probably at work. He had the further bad luck of being sick enough that nobody was entirely sure which way this was going to go.

What no one had explicitly said out loud, but some of my colleagues seemingly believed, was that he wouldn't be in this mess if he just had the good sense to slim down. I mean, he's a doctor, treating people with diabetes and heart attacks for heaven's sake, surely he knows the risks? Between the long days and night shifts, with their attendant microwave meals and cortisol spikes, could he not go for a run and have a salad? Judging by my diet and sloth-like exercise regimen over the past month, I wouldn't be so sure. In reality, his body shape was as much the outcome of a genetic roulette wheel as an indication of willpower.

Even if this was all his fault, there wasn't much he could do now. I completed the pain-in-the-arse process of safely layering up, before stepping into the (hopefully) hermetically sealed bay.

Whoever thought heroism would involve wearing two hair nets and a pair of sweat-steeped communal wellies?

This side of the hospital was being cooked by the early summer sun, everyone in the bay cursing the uncharacteristically panoramic windows. There was no air conditioning, and it was impossible to know if this was a safety thing, to avoid circulating infected air, or just because no one wanted to pay for it. The resulting heat turned the inside into a toxic greenhouse.

Standing in front of him, the face shield reinforced the distance between us. He was on 60 per cent oxygen through a CPAP (continuous positive airway pressure) machine and had a lot of extra pressure blowing into his face to encourage his airways to open. If we had to turn either of the dials up further, then we were heading for tube time. One problem with having a doctor as your patient is it's very difficult to bullshit them.

'How am I doing?'

'Well at least everything's stable.'

'Being stably *terrible* is not a good thing.'

'Yes, true . . . but at least you're not any *more* terrible than when I saw you this morning.'

'It's . . . easy to be . . . optimistic when you're not the one in this box . . . watching your neighbours dragged off in a coma . . . or dead.'

I didn't have an adequate response for this, so decided to exercise one of the powers I did have – to make an excuse and leave.

'Let me go and find out from the lab how long your blood results will be.'

With that, I scuttled away, my smooth exit hampered by the complicated PPE removal at the door to the bay. I sat at a computer, looking for bloods I knew wouldn't be back, to at least maintain some veneer of truth to my words.

He wasn't the only staff member to have gotten sick, here or anywhere. More of them have names closer to Omar than Geoff or Tristan. The elevated position of doctor is no guarantee, never fully insulates you from the racial inequities in society. Studies in America have demonstrated poorer health among wealthy black individuals even compared to their poor white counterparts. Inequity can bind an ankle like seaweed, pulling you back under as you grasp at the shore.

With deaths among healthcare workers, particularly doctors, the figures are even more skewed relative to the general population: at least 85 per cent of healthcare worker COVID deaths were from ethnic minority backgrounds. Early in the pandemic, 95 per cent of doctors who died were non-white (as compared to 51 per cent of all junior doctors and 41 per cent of consultants). Despite having attained a level of relative prosperity, they have retained some disadvantage – one that traverses generations, pulling that newly purchased expensive rug from under their feet.

They are more likely to have spent their early lives in less advantageous conditions, with the associated stresses and lifetime health effects. They may also be supporting a wider network of dependents and family members, impacting how and when they work, taking on more physically harmful shift patterns.

There is growing interest in the possibility that stressful life events alter the genetic material passed on to offspring, with DNA modifications switching genes off and on, potentially providing further reasons the socially mobile may not be able to escape the health issues that affect other, less fortunate members of their ethnic group.

As much as it's easy to stray into dodgy territory when considering genetic causes of health inequalities, looking at the more important social and public health determinants can be equally fertile soil for awful takes. Practices and beliefs can be maliciously presented as evidence of some cultural inferiority, rather than traditions that are simply ill-suited to the current situation. Circumstances, such as living in overcrowded accommodation, become more than just the product of opportunity (or lack thereof).

It's vital to determine the underlying causes of differing outcomes, but in a way that retains sensitivity, and without judgement. Inevitably this will come from involving people in research that is about them, and having a genuine desire to progress towards equity underpinning all such work.

CHAPTER 11

Putting the 'Fun' in 'Funeral'

THE ROLLOUT CONTINUED – on what seemed like a daily basis we would come in to find a new space had been designated as medical beds, now someone's additional responsibility. This week, it was the gastrointestinal and bariatric surgical ward – almost all but their most emergency work had been cancelled (it's bad form to kill someone with hospital-acquired COVID in the pursuit of their bariatric weight-loss goals). And we needed the space. Given the restrictions on travel, the beach body and eventual reduced cardiovascular risk could wait.

In an older part of the hospital, the decor and upholstery hadn't been updated since the 1990s at best. There was a general QVC look to the place. All of the hard surfaces were a cream off-white, the floor deep green vinyl.

Today I was the HDU outreach registrar, which meant combing through the list of patients flagged for review, making what felt like only one decision: CPAP yes or no. It seemed to be working for some patients, keeping them off a ventilator, or useful as a last resort, if they weren't fit enough to survive a visit from the tube team. I had been asked to come and see someone who on paper sounded like he was in trouble.

Around him was a sea of silver, but despite being 80, Mr Levy retained a suspiciously deep oil-slick black swoop of a mane. Vanity can be a life-saver – it made him look ten years younger than the others, and at a time when snap decisions based on age and perceived frailty seemed rife, this could make all the difference.

He was alert and good-humoured – but tired. By the standards of other illnesses, however, he didn't look nearly as endangered as the numbers on his monitor suggested. The reading from the sats probe was bouncing up and down the scale, but would dip as low as the 70s, despite the oxygen being cranked to the maximum on the wall. He was breathing quickly, and the star of David pendant that nestled in the snow-flecked thicket of his chest hair emphasised the movement.

'How are you feeling, Mr Levy?'

'I tell you what . . . this has really knocked me for six.'

'I'm not surprised – your oxygen levels are so low I'm amazed you're able to talk.'

'I'm a cab driver – it'll take more than this to shut me up.'

I hope I'm able to be like this – able to laugh even with the spectre in the room. Then again, I'm certain my family will have long tired of my brand of 'humour' and will be pushing the oxygen mask back onto my face for a little peace.

'I'm here to see if you need to come to the high-dependency unit for some extra help.'

'And what sort of help . . . *can* you give me? Apparently I'm in a bit of a pickle.'

'Well, we would fit a mask over your face – it pushes air into your lungs to help you breathe.'

'So you're going to save my life with a hairdryer?'

'You could say that . . . although it's not how they put it in the textbook.'

'What are my odds with it . . . compared to without it?'

'It's really hard to say – but this is the last thing we have left to offer, and it's your best chance.'

He was 80, with a significant smoking history and oxygen levels that should have rendered him unconscious, so those chances definitely weren't good either way.

'If I'm being honest, I'm knackered. What's it like – is it uncomfortable?'

'Well at first it's not the most . . . pleasant feeling – but lots of people get used to it eventually.'

'You're really selling it to me . . . and the ward, is it noisy? It might seem like . . . I love the sound of my own voice, but . . . I just want some peace.'

I was taken aback by him weighing up like this, but he was far more astute than others in his situation. If I were going to die either way, the demented fairground of beeps that can be a critical care environment wouldn't be my first choice either.

'Let me speak to my wife – but I'm not sure I'm up for it.'

'Okay – but the longer we leave it, the worse it will get.'

I left him with the curtains around his bed and the uneasy feeling that in all likelihood he wouldn't be coming, and would take his chances out here in the relative tranquillity, away from the cacophony.

* * *

On the HDU, the inevitable had happened. We were hosting four times the number of patients we would have under normal circumstances. They were housed in a series of walled-off, four-bed boxes, receiving near-identical treatment.

I had admitted Mr Shah almost two weeks previously, when my job had been waving the coughing masses into the hospital. His medical rap sheet was an instant heart sink – suffering from idiopathic pulmonary fibrosis, an absolute arsehole of a condition, in which inflammation gradually gnarls and scars lung tissue for no clear good reason.

If I were ever so unlucky, the kicker for me would be the word 'idiopathic' – to be slowly killed by something so vague that the collective medical wisdom had nothing better to call it than the linguistic equivalent of a shrug. The steroids used over the years to rescue him from flare-ups and prevent further damage to his lungs had accelerated his type-2 diabetes. Both of these together put a target on his back when it came to COVID.

I hadn't held out much hope for him lasting the night he came in, but had neglected to follow up and confirm my fears once he had been absorbed and sunk into the morass of admissions. I was uncharacteristically happy at being proved incorrect when I found him chugging away on the newly commissioned, rheumatology-staffed COVID ward a week later. I usually hate being wrong, but even I will make an excuse for occasions when patients outlive my pessimism. My joy was brief, however, as it soon became apparent that he wasn't doing well.

He had remained stuck, with little improvement in spite of time and oxygen – the two things that were making patients better. Though only in his 50s, his crater-marked lungs made him a terrible candidate for ventilation. The only option, then, was CPAP as a final Hail Mary. When I rotated onto the HDU for my on-calls, and encountered him for the third time, I learned that this hadn't hit the mark. The flight mask-like apparatus was off, and he was being 'kept comfortable'. This phrase, 'comfort', is so frequently a prelude to the end, stalking the corridors of the hospital, it's enough to give you a phobia of soft furnishings and loungewear, but under these circumstances it's among the most vital things we do.

Over several hours he had gradually become less responsive, until finally drifting off completely. In the bay, from behind the glass, before the curtains were closed, he looked like Lenin in his tomb, as if just resting, eyes closed. One of the FY1s had done the job of confirming and the nurses had spoken to his family, so there wasn't anything left to do.

This was just the beginning, however. After being whisked off to the hospital basement, the Byzantine process of getting him buried would begin. Patient affairs and the mortuary are, under normal circumstances, primed to expedite things for Muslim, and indeed Orthodox Jewish families, to enable funerals to take place as soon as possible. At the height of the pandemic, with more work coupled with the need for infection control, this was unlikely.

Families waited days, sometimes weeks, to receive loved ones, causing more distress. Around half waited longer than three weeks before a service could take place. Even more painfully, those who had chosen to be with their relatives at the end in person were then forced to isolate for 14 days. If by some cruel irony the process then ran smoothly, this quarantine and the date of the funeral would overlap, and they would be unable to attend.

Send-offs were depressing, even by normal morbid standards. Zoom funerals, among the bleakest of word fusions, became a reality. Mourners were forced to pay their respects from the confines of tiny grief windows, peering out from the wall of sorrow, trying to resist the urge to catch up on some email admin mid-service.

* * *

Some funeral traditions have had further to fall to reach their pandemic-mandated nadirs than others. The Church of England could learn a little from my aunt's pre-COVID service at the Kingdom of Heaven Baptist Church, Birmingham after she died at 57 from a vanishingly rare disease, the kind of medical curiosity that had no doubt gotten her medical team *very* excited. This was a direct and painful reminder of the personal story underlying every diagnostic curiosity.

From the outside, the venue was an inauspicious-looking, single-storey concrete cube on the edge of an industrial estate – apparently the lord and saviour had stuck to his modest biblical roots when house hunting. Mourners' cars vied for space with tradesmen visiting Screwfix.

Aside from the demographics, the most noticeable difference compared to the *Songs of Praise* crowd, there was a band. Not some low-key source of sombre ambiance, but a group complete with a drummer, two guitarists and bass, who looked and sounded like they were aiming to resurrect Luther Vandross there and then. We were spared the dirge of C of E hymns – the kind that start every bar with a slurred drone from the organ in an effort to give the congregation time to stumble into sync, but with the end result sounding like the groans of distressed cattle.

They were already playing as we walked in, soundtracking the awkward few seconds as the ushers calculated where we qualified to sit. Weddings and funerals, the occasions we get to see our rank in the emotional league table. This time, second row (not bad considering my dad's wealth of siblings and the number of cousins that followed).

We were handed orders of service, and the 1980s and 90s came alive in the family photos that were included in the gloss pages of the booklet. As is often the case, grief's companion was nostalgia – briefly nudged from sorrow by a glimpse of the brown-orange patterned carpet in Nan's good front room, a 70s relic, and the plastic that remained permanently on the sofas.

Aside from the musicians, the stage was packed. The pastor had a bigger entourage than your favourite rapper – and it was equally difficult to discern what everyone was doing up there. A particular oddity was the lone white face in the choir, a grey-suited man in his sixties, with his serious expression looking like an accountant who had gotten lost, wandered into a congregation and in a panic picked up a tambourine.

Important attendees were introduced by name: Bishop Lewis from the nearby New Glory Holy Trinity Church had magnanimously graced us with his presence, despite the unclear personal relationship. For church dignitaries, funerals are perhaps the equivalent of a local celebrity's supermarket ribbon cutting.

No matter how packed the stage, the role of hype man is already taken in black Pentecostal churches. In the hip-hop world, touring excesses and insufficient cardio mean MCs usually need a couple of buddies to finish every other line, and hand them white towels. The pastor has the church ladies. They're ready with the ad-libs, and can time a 'Praise Jesus' better than Migos could time a 'Skrrt skrrt' (this is the most current hip-hop reference you're getting from me).

The band quietened to a simmer and the pastor began in an accent that wandered from Birmingham UK to Birmingham Alabama.

'We are here to bid farewell to our sister – as she leaves, to sit at the side of our lord in heaven. Now did he not promise us that he was the word?'

'Yes he did.'

'And if we listened to the word, we would be granted eternity at his side in paradise?'

This was greeted with widespread affirmation by the audience: 'Mmhhmm.'

Every rhetorical device that formed the scaffolding of the great American civil rights speech was recognisable, reclaimed to support its original, holy purpose. It was around the time the band stirred back up they really got to me. Sure, you may think you're a hyper-rational man of science, immune to more spiritual powers. I walked in secure in my heathenistic lack of belief and by the end, as the four-to-the-floor kickdrum of 'Every Praise' hit, I was practically shopping for a tambourine to match the accountant's on Amazon.

This effect was fleeting; the only time you'll catch me at a church service is when someone gets married or dies. Nevertheless, it can't be argued with: in my limited experience, black churches are far from dull, home to a spirit with the power to grab you, and singing that doesn't make you curse the gift of hearing.

When he had finished, and the band had played us out, we drove the short distance to the cemetery, for the moment that feels truly final. It's a scene you might imagine rendered cliched by film, but, if anything, the familiarity, the routine of the final farewell, focuses and distils the emotion. You know the rhythms, anticipate the beats, guided how to feel and when.

After the immortal words reminding us to where we must return were spoken, and the box lowered, the assembled took turns throwing in a handful of soil. Caught up, I joined, scrabbling over a mound of dirt in my suit and brogues. A respectable distance away, two young men, cemetery employees, stood looking solemnly impatient next to the digger that would shift the final earth.

After the service and committal, the wake served the secondary, conciliatory purpose that was denied so many during the pandemic. It brought together a family that have been flung far and wide by the practicalities of trying to forge a life. I have enough cousins to lose track, and this was the first time we had all been in the same place for years.

The pastor was there, too, though I'm not sure if this is the norm. The one key difference being that, out of his vestments, he was back to being just my uncle Michael. By day, he does something in computing I confess I have failed to commit to memory, but by night he works for a higher power. How he navigated overseeing his own, closest sister's funeral, and kept it together, I will never fully comprehend.

The event was hardly sombre, and in some ways felt closer to a wedding reception. I mean, there was a DJ, something I have never seen before or since at a funeral (I'm not sure of the most appropriate number of air horn blasts for this sort of occasion).

Despite spending her entire career as a social worker, my Aunt Odette's true calling is clearly feeding on a grand scale. Having taken charge of the organising, she had managed to sort catering for the upwards of 150 people who came. There was curry goat, brown stewed chicken and rice and peas, all steaming in giant silver vats. It was a spread to inspire funeral crashing, spurious connections concocted in the hope of a plate.

This was the sort of event that carried the constant risk of social awkwardness. The face of a member of my dad's generation could suddenly appear, beaming, leaving me scrabbling to hide that I had no idea who this distant relative or friend was. There would be much nodding and pretending to remember anecdotes from a time before I was even old enough to form memories. On the plus side, no one squeezed my cheek.

A reminder of the pull of working life on a family, I wasn't able to stay for long – having to leave Birmingham that evening. I had to get back for an on-call shift that started early the following day. At least in a family that almost fetishises working in medicine, this obligation was understood.

That such gatherings were denied so many, although necessary, is a loss that can't be undone. For the few able to attend gatherings, singing was banned – songs of praise spraying aerosols too much of a risk. No wake, whether with cold sandwiches or curry. No chance to get together and share the weight of the loss.

CHAPTER 12

Learn the Lingo

SITTING AT THE MDF and plastic desk in the resuscitation area, or 'resus', three computers are fought over by four times as many doctors and nurses. They swarm in and around, darting when they see an opening – a colleague forced to vacate prime real estate by an alarm sounding from their patient's monitor. At least the burden of phone calls, bleeps and the sacred task of maintaining the take list mean once I'm there, I'm fixed, limpet-like for the foreseeable.

The only windows are meagre vents high in the utility-grey walls. It certainly never feels like daylight, since any that creeps in is bleached out by the icy LEDs overhead. The timelessness has its advantages, allowing you to forget what the hospital is keeping you from. It's not your best friend's wedding, or simply the last good day of summer – just another 12 hours. Now at least the level of FOMO is limited, since, for the most part, friends are spending their days careering between baking, day drinking and repentant exercise.

Other than intensive care, this is where the sickest patients are, or at least where they should be, when there's space. This is the COVID side of ED, and it's a full house. The red ambulance phone menaces on the desk. If it follows through with the threat and rings, the message 'respiratory blue call, ten minutes' will mean time for us to do some shuffling. Not that any of the patients we already have on deck are necessarily well or stable enough to be booted out. Fortunately, for now, it holds fire – so we only teeter on the edge of calamity, rather than plunging in.

When the hospital is full, waiting for space to free up is essentially hoping that the happier of the two possible outcomes happens downstream, clearing the log jam – namely that someone leaves the hospital alive, freeing up a bed, rather than . . . the alternative. Then again, you very rarely get to find out which it actually is.

The view from behind the nurses' station is surreal. The ten beds housed in individual glass-fronted recesses look like tanks in an aquarium. Inside each, a patient engages in the same struggle – getting enough oxygen. Some sit oblivious, calm despite their worrying vitals, with 'happy hypoxia'. Others gasp like fish out of water, all too aware of their predicament.

Our options are limited in this situation. Once you've turned up the oxygen as far as it goes and tried a bit of 'proning' (putting the patient on their front to help their lungs expand, aka 'tummy time'), you're left waiting. Waiting either for them to get better, or for anaesthetics to come along and say yay or nay to putting a tube down Mrs Madhvani's throat to help her breathe. This medicine is at once some of the simplest and most difficult I have done.

Many families among the large South Asian population in the local area are close, with several generations often living under the same roof. She has been on hand, giving her children the most precious gift of all (after life itself): free babysitting, witnessing milestones in her grandchildren's lives she would have missed in the confines of a euphemistically titled 'retirement community'. In return, her kids pay her in kind, ferrying her to see friends and her ever-multiplying hospital appointments.

Among the worst is trying to remember and then explain today's restrictions. Last I checked, one family member can visit before they go under, but I can't be 100 per cent certain the pestilent wind hasn't changed, and the rules with it, in the last five minutes. Whatever, for now Mrs Madhvani's daughter is in the room with her mother, swaddled in PPE, gripping her hand and begging her to hold on. They both have the same, searing ice-blue-grey eyes I can still see now.

My usefulness exhausted, I sit uncharacteristically idle when I get a call through the switchboard from outside the hospital. It's a psychotically chirpy oncology registrar, asking if we might be able to check over one of his patients who is feeling unwell at home after their recent chemotherapy.

The reason some patients feel unwell is that, in trying to smoke out the cancer, oncologists end up napalming a lot of good stuff in the process. Good stuff including the immune system. Given the viral miasma floating around, ED is currently a place where a functional immune system is one of 'this season's must-haves'. I point this out to him.

There isn't a great deal he can say to this. Although they do seem to have a knack for occasionally bringing their patients tantalisingly close, oncologists tend to have a real aversion to them actually dying. It's not unheard of for some to balk when the palliative care team broach that it may be time to let someone go. An old joke, which I will shamelessly regurgitate, goes:

'How many oncologists do you need to be pallbearers at a funeral? Five. That's four to carry the casket, and one to hang the chemo.'

Not that I blame them – they're often the last lifeline keeping patients suspended above the void. Even when it goes well it can be an under-recognised job. To many patients, the people with the knives wield the cure: 'Thanks to my amazing surgeon, getting the whole tumour, clear margins, I'm still here.' The oncologist, on the other hand, just made them sick.

I look at the full spaces and heaving list in front of me. For once, my overwhelming desire not to add to my workload has aligned with what's best for the patient. We agree to try to find a plan B, one that doesn't involve bringing them here and killing them in the process. Just before I put the phone down, I ask him to remind me of his name, and process it properly for the first time. His voice suddenly clicks in my head. I had worked with him when he was a hot-off-the-production-line FY1 and I was an FY2, but he had arrived looking ready for the private clinic–golf course axis. Some reflex causes my voice to climb a couple of privilege rungs.

'Toby, I haven't spoken to you for ages! How's it going? Pre-pandemic, every picture you posted, you looked like you had just stepped off a yacht.'

'Yes, well unfortunately it looks like those days are behind me for now.'

'And *that* is the real tragedy of this all, never mind all the, you know . . . death. Still, I'm sure you'll be back in St Tropez in no time.'

'How posh do you think I am?'

'Do you really want me to answer that question? I bet you're wearing boat shoes right now.'

(A brief silence.) 'Touché.'

'And speaking French – see.'

I hang up the phone, ignorant of the fact that, as well as getting posher, I have become several decibels louder, as is customary among such people. I notice Marta, one of the nurses looking at me sceptically.

'Did you go to private school?'

'Err no, why?'

'Because you certainly *sound* like it.'

She is of course right. While I hardly sounded like Oliver Twist as a child, medicine has filed down any rough edges there were, leaving a perfectly smooth replica public-school plum. Originally from Poland, working in ED alongside junior doctors has given Marta a crash course in the English class system – watching middle- and upper middle-class doctors collide with the wider world, the cotton wool they grew up wrapped in now soaked in the blood and piss of uncoddled reality.

* * *

Unfair as it is, being able to code-switch when needed is arguably a key life skill – up there with numeracy and being able to tie one's own shoelaces. In the absence of long-overdue societal overhaul, you could envisage teaching it in state schools, for the sake of social mobility.

Like many men now in early middle age, moaning about the state of modern hip-hop, I grew up wishing I sounded like a member of the Wu-Tang Clan. A glimmer of self-awareness, however, and a desire not to get beaten or laughed to a pulp, meant I never ambled too far down that path. I was from Catford, not Staten Island, and what's more, I went to a nice middle-class school in Bromley. And then there was my dad.

Speaking 'properly' was important to him. It's how you make

the world listen. If you ever 'aksed' him for something, not only would you not get it, but instead you would be the recipient of a short seminar on how language is key to getting ahead in life. His slow, deliberate Trevor McDonald tones are the result of an over-correction – speech lessons to overcome a stammer, his aunt's insistence on all things proper, coupled with the transfer from Jamaica to a 1960s Britain educational system – one still plenty hostile to any linguistic flavour imported from the colonies.

Jamaica is a small foot that has made a big cultural print, something every other island in the Caribbean is sick of hearing about. Still, no Jamaica, no Kool Herc moving to the Bronx, no hip-hop. 'Bad' would still just mean bad. Closer to home, few who speak the dialect ever called it 'Multicultural London English', but whatever name you give it, a lot of what I heard in the Lewisham playgrounds of the 1990s was as Jamaican as the bass vibrating the speakers of passing cars.

As quickly as marginalised youth can come up with music and a sub-culture, suburbia will sanitise it and absorb the elements it likes. As long as the kids don't talk like that at the dinner table, or in a job interview, it's all good. This isn't how the doctors of tomorrow speak when it really matters – heaven forbid people be treated by someone who sounds like them.

This conflict hasn't been without a cost. In some ways, it has rendered me a tourist to my own home culture. Ask me to speak with a Jamaican accent and you'll be disappointed, then beg me to stop. The best you'll get is a paper-thin caricature, easily buffeted from passable to outright offensive.

The same doesn't go for everyone in my extended family, but as well as being linguistically distant, they live in Birmingham, basically another country. I won't mire myself in the cliche of claiming not to have an accent – my southern, mainly Received

Pronunciation is just the least interesting possible, making it much easier to shed. As a child, five minutes around my cousins and I ripped off this stiff uniform and swapped it for what felt like a cape. This new Brumaican was of course met with bemusement and ridicule on my return to south-east London and quickly put away, eventually to be lost entirely, but while I had it, it fit perfectly.

University finished the job, since despite whatever success there may have been in widening access, medical school was still full of private-school kids. Their confident, chummy braying reverberated through the halls and lecture theatres. They all co-opted the word 'mate' and everything was 'banter'. A person could even *be* banter – Chris is good banter, Vicky is bad banter. Inevitably said banter seemed to involve drinking to the point of alcohol poisoning, for reasons loosely related to sport, being punished for losing drinking games everyone seemed to have learned at boarding school. Apparently, the old boys network was to be cemented by the rugby team sitting in a circle vomiting into bin liners.

Reading textbooks, there were times I lamented not having a public-school education. You learn an incredible number of new words studying medicine – but if you did Latin and Greek at school, you have one hell of a head start, since that's the language the 19th-century gentleman physicians chose when naming everything. Boris Johnson would barely have to look anything up. Then again, what helps in the classroom is likely to bamboozle patients and need translating back into plain English anyway (not that doctors have cared too much about that in the past), so *item et ambages* – or 'swings and roundabouts' according to Google Translate.

As a patient, how you speak may save your life. 'Well-spoken' native English speakers often get better treatment – healthcare workers subconsciously aware that the sharpened middle-class elbow is the last thing you want digging into your career. You never know – they could be a lawyer; they might golf with the local MP. You could be one bad consultation away from calamity. Better instead to roll out the red carpet and genuflect appropriately.

For the rest, the hospital is a foreign land with a strange language, one that appears constructed to empower doctors and obfuscate what a patient really wants to know. We love a euphemism. Just try getting a doctor to say the word 'cancer' up front. You can't; instead we say we're doing scans 'just to check there's nothing sinister', like we're worried it's going to reveal a picture of Nigel Farage's face underneath the skin.

Medical specialties name themselves to feel clever – and to ensure you know they are too. You go to see your cardiologist, respiratory physician and ophthalmologist, not your heart, lung and eye doctors. And as I've already complained, almost no one knows what rheumatology is. I can't think of any other reason to persist with this. It doesn't help anyone else.

Doctors from different specialties also all speak differently, depending on the balance of action and intellect we want to project into the world. Ever dynamic, I remember one hot-blooded cardiologist who would never image the blood vessels in your heart, but rather 'shoot your coronaries'. And why would I ever say a patient has come in with cold symptoms, when I can proudly exclaim he has 'coryza'? Much more impressive.

At your appointment, God help you if you have any trouble with English. Things have gotten better, but in the past you were lucky if you were offered a translator. Apparently the hope being that you wouldn't know to ask for one – with the plan instead that the consultation would be conducted as a very high-stakes game of charades, praying you wouldn't need to act out gastroenteritis.

If you *do* get a translator, they almost certainly won't be in the room with you, but rather on the end of a phone. Now, this can work fine, but often it doesn't. I have had many circular, increasingly baffling conversations that as they spiralled left me dizzy, with a worse headache than the patient. There is no extra time allocated to deal with this added barrier between us and excavating the root of their problem. As the clinic backs up behind the impasse, we find ourselves wrapping up a consultation having achieved next to nothing, everyone more confused than when they came in.

Some of us take matters into our own hands. Dr Sharp, my boss at the Trench (as a reminder, a white man from one of the less ethnically diverse parts of the UK), has learned so many Gujarati and Punjabi words that Shivani, one of the other registrars, felt embarrassed by comparison: 'Dr Sharp is a better brown person than I am! I can barely string two words together when I try.'

Needs must. It was certainly preferable to sitting opposite the patient, both staring at each other in silence, or relying entirely on the prism-like effect of the accompanying relative's translation, notorious for refracting and scattering the truth in subtle but important ways.

Still, a little knowledge can be a dangerous thing, and is easily misused. In areas with large Bangladeshi populations, staff have familiarised themselves with the word 'bish' – meaning 'pain' in Sylheti (unsurprisingly a pretty common complaint in an emergency department). Accompanying this knowledge, however, has been the idea among some doctors that older, female patients from this group complain of symptoms like 'whole body bish' (sometimes offensively labelled 'Bibi syndrome'), and that it is often of psychological, rather than physical, origin. Although this may be the cause in some cases, as with any group, it is unhelpful, given that this is also a cohort disproportionately likely to have heart attacks – and their coronary arteries aren't blocked with feelings.

* * *

The cavalry has arrived for bed six. Although they could be here for any of them; my charges are all on their list. The anaesthetists arrive en-masse, the action shifting to slow-mo as they stride over the resus threshold. The drama is heightened by the full-hooded respirator the consultant is forced to wear, because his face is just simply too big, chiselled and masculine to fit a conventional FFP3 mask. In the white helmet, he looks ready to traverse the surface of an alien planet.

Before they brave entering the room, they huddle and go round the circle, reminding everyone what their jobs will be once inside – as if they could have forgotten, having done this too many times today already. Satisfied, they head in, ushering out Mrs Madhvani's tearful daughter.

As they work, we gawp through the glass, eyes darting between the movement of their hands and the pulse oximeter numbers.

'How many anaesthetists does it take to screw in an ET tube?' Marta chimes.

'Three of them, and a nurse apparently.'

Infantry always gripes about the prima donnas when they ride to the rescue on horseback. We're just jealous really. Historically, anaesthetics have been one of the few specialities who have convinced hospital management to let them have a safe number of staff to do their jobs properly – at least before the pandemic. We resent them for this luxury. Then again, if they mess up, failing to get oxygen into the comatose individual in front of them, people can die pretty quickly – often young people, so probably for the best.

My eyes fix on the saturation monitor, hypnotised by the serene, undulating blue trace – a sinusoidal comfort blanket. When everything goes to plan, anaesthetics is all about calm, even when doing things that would make us mere mortals incontinent with fear. What I can tell you about the procedure will be limited, since whenever anyone tries to talk in too much depth about 'the science bit' of anaesthetics, I glaze over slightly. Not that I'm not interested in the physiology – it's just usually delivered in the context of them telling you for the 100th time how reassuringly difficult their specialty exams are.

Among the jargon I have ignored, I have heard the term 'rapid sequence induction' bandied about, and they seemed to be inducing anaesthesia rapidly, so let's go with that. After the sleepy juice has gone into the vein, along with the paralysis agent, the patient derelicts the duty of breathing for themselves pretty quickly. It's vital, then, that something is done to rectify this situation soon – namely connecting the ventilator. An assistant will have been diligently 'bagging' the patient – ensuring as much air as possible gets in before the safety harness is detached and the breathless highwire act can begin.

Almost no sound escapes the hermetic seal of the room. I watch the silent thriller of a life-and-death mime show. The mask comes away and the sickled blade of the laryngoscope slides over the tongue, to be wedged into the vallecula (ridge at the back of the tongue) allowing the glottis (hole between the vocal cords) to be visualised – at least when things go to plan. A lot of anatomy learning, several new words and careful practice go into intubation – what is essentially putting one tube into another, slightly larger tube. Even then, there are no guarantees in an emergency – just the hope that the forward yank reveals a clear path. The plastic pipe hangs interminably in the consultant's hand, then an abrupt shift and it is desperately stuffed along the steel guide wire. In place and quickly married with the ventilator, 21 cm of plastic becomes a breath-fogged lifeline.

Mrs Madhvani's chest rises and falls, and the drama recedes. The more mundane tasks take over – connecting the mobile monitor, making sure she is untethered from the resus bay, and a half-hearted attempt to make sure her property makes the journey with her upstairs to ITU. If she awakens and the biggest problem is a misplaced pair of glasses, I think we could consider that a win.

The doors part and she is wheeled away, the process transitioning her from being my most pressing concern to a phantom. Statistically, her fate is now a coin toss I no longer have any means of influencing. I'll be left to remotely pry into the ITU notes to find out which way it lands.

CHAPTER 13

Elective Work

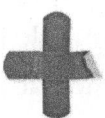

AROUND HOSPITALS, SOMETHING that had quickly fallen by the wayside was clinical teaching. A procession of eager ears leaning over a patient to listen to their fragile heart, in the hope of hearing some exciting murmur – and in the process risking infecting them, or vice versa, was hard to justify. But in many cases, the medical students were still there.

Many of them had answered the call to help. They were on the wards doing everything from restocking cupboards, moving patients and, yes, that often-disregarded task of helping cleaning and wiping patients. This was a far cry from my memory of the final year of medical school, which, aside from the small issue of exams (assuming all went to plan), at times felt like a victory lap. This cohort weren't going to their last university parties, weren't sneaking in a last trip abroad, if they could afford it, before being made slaves to the rota.

This nostalgia for university is of course only possible because the memory has been cleansed of so much anxiety. The version of yourself you look back on is no longer weighed by the nagging fear of how things will turn out, whether you will be a success. Gone also is the worry that you're not quite at the centre of things, the event you should be at, the perfect night out – the feeling of chasing a carnival procession that's always a street away, no matter how quickly you race towards the sound of the music.

Inevitably some overcompensate, coming across as impossibly confident. They have a destabilising certainty about how the world works, and what they're going to do in it. A conversation with one of these self-assured young men at one of those aforementioned parties comes to mind.

'And of course the little buggers live in the reeds on the banks of Lake Malawi – so you just have to neck some Praziquantel every now and then, because it's hardly like you're *not* going to swim in bloody Lake Malawi.'

This bore had been talking to me about snails, the parasites they harbour (the same critters that would one day nearly derail my doctor–patient relationship with Mr Maseko on cardiology) and his *Lonely Planet* adventures for the last 15 minutes. He was one of the more trying species of medical students – the budding international infectious diseases guy. The pathology manifests as a more extreme variety of the kid who arrives at university and makes their gap year their whole personality – he wanted to spin it out into an entire career, but with limited insight into what the job actually entails.

'Is there much call for tropical snail parasite remedies in London, where you live and presumably are going to have to treat patients?'

He scoffed at this.

'I'll be out of the country most of the time anyway – yeah, basically I'll do an ACF, train in ID and then do a lot of MSF.'

He had certainly perfected the acronym salad (Academic Clinical Fellowship, Infectious Diseases and Médecins Sans Frontières, in case you're wondering). The confidence was almost admirable – 150 years ago he'd probably have been dressed in khaki, regaling cocktail parties with tales of his most recent ivory expedition over a gin and tonic (quinine to keep the malaria at bay). He probably couldn't wait to wow us with the Swahili he learned building wells in Kenya on his gap year.

Funnily, most of his humanitarian zeal was directed towards places where you can top up your tan. It was tempting to quiz him about something closer to home, given the reality for many infection doctors working in the UK is diagnosing the motley crew of bugs making a leg ulcer reek, and negotiating with heroin users to take their endocarditis antibiotics without nipping off the ward to shoot up (which can be a tall order, given the cannula we so kindly insert helpfully doubles as the perfect smack delivery system).

Every once in a while, there *is* the excitement of a fever in a returning traveller, the opportunity to nose into the sweaty recesses of their recent past – which part of the country they trekked to, what they ate and who they slept with when they were there. Of course, often it's just malaria – frequently someone born in west Africa, assuming because they never had to take prophylaxis growing up, they'll be fine on their travels home. Little do they know that, living in England, their idle and pampered immune system has grown soft, and any immunity earned throughout childhood has waned.

Mastery of the art of exiting a conversation like this is vital – you have to sense the motion and catch the wave that's going to propel you out of it and back to shore. Even better if you can find a float in the form of someone you'd rather be talking to –

or you can at the very least palm this jerk off to. I spotted my chance as two friendlier faces drifted past from the kitchen.

'Paul, Rachel, have you met James? You really must . . . And anyway I just need to go and get a drink.'

And before the poor unsuspecting fools realised what was happening, I was away, and they were left to be swallowed up by the tide of inane chat.

Rescued, I found Tommy on the other side of the living room.

'Where have you been?'

'I got stuck talking to Captain Colonial.'

I can't take credit for this nickname – it was originally coined by Osman, one of the few male students who took the Global Health intercalated BSc who didn't match the description of private-school boy with a saviour complex.

'How have you managed to come to a party and find yourself getting a live recitation of the *Heart of Darkness*?'

The irony is, most medical students have a pretty poor idea of what they 'want to do when they grow up', as it's often patronisingly put by their seniors. As well as training in emergency medicine, Tommy would end up volunteering in Sudan, Kenya and refugee camps on the Greek islands – but at least he has the good graces to shut up about it every once in a while. He is far more likely to bore you talking about wine terroir than remedies for parasitic illnesses.

None of this is to put down my current infectious diseases colleagues (which might make the next time I ask them for help investigating a fever of unknown origin a little awkward). I find with maturity and experience of the job, comes some perspective, and the ability to tone it all down a bit. There is also the obvious counterpoint, that as sceptical as I may want to be about the altruistic motives of others, my contribution to improving the lives of those in tropical and other developing countries is precisely zero.

The crowning moment of medical school for the explorer medic (and to be honest for the vast majority of us) is the elective. In the final year, all students are given the opportunity to spend eight weeks focused on an area of medicine of their choosing. Crucially, this can be anywhere in the world – some squares travel to an illustrious neurosurgery programme in peak Boston winter. There they are flogged like American medical students, in the hope that it will improve their chances of someday being allowed to take power tools to some poor soul's skull.

Others see this as the opportunity it really is: for eight weeks of barely supervised fun on the other side of the world – preferably somewhere near the equator and with a coastline. There is the small matter of being 'signed off' at the end – the host institution rubber-stamping the fact you actually showed up. Don't take the piss, show your face enough that they at least recognise you when waving the form under their nose, and you'll probably be fine. In any case, the pandemic iced this particular opportunity for a sizeable cohort of students.

* * *

I'm not a natural-born traveller – my desire for comfort and familiarity extends to more than just an aversion to camping. My compulsion to avoid danger also means I'm loath to expose myself to chaotic roads and angry fauna. Still, part of me realised the elective probably wasn't an opportunity to be passed up, so with no ideas of my own, I tagged onto the trip to Samoa that Tommy was planning with Kyron and some other friends from football – I would be the token non-sportsman.

Samoa (pronounced 'Saar-moa' if you're from there, or

the type of person who returns from their travels obnoxiously intent on letting everyone know they've soaked up the culture) ticked all of my boxes on the safety front. Too sleepy for roads to be that lethal, as I write it's officially malaria-free, and the only real poisonous creature mentioned in the guidebooks is a rare sea snail – which even with my lack of pace I think I could outrun.

After a truly pointless 20-hour stopover in New Zealand, we stepped off the modern but conspicuously small plane into the greenhouse heat of a Pacific Island tropical paradise, the aesthetic so much the ideal, it almost looked computer-rendered. In Apia, the capital, we would do the month or so of actual work and learning that would justify our jaunt around the world. I chose to split my time between paediatrics and adult general medicine. Ward rounds for the latter were led by Dr Keil, a quiet man whose patience our group truly tested while there.

Tall, broad and with a face that looked hewn from Samoan rock, he often found himself with the pleasure of our physical, if not mental, presence. He eschewed scrubs in favour of the traditional kilt-like lavalava and a shirt, methodically plodding through the patients on the ward, flip-flops slapping as he went.

'And what class of antiarrhythmic is amiodarone?'

He scanned the blank faces of the British cohort, his optimism shifting quickly to disappointment. He had come to learn about us, that having access to the shiniest London hospitals won't make you actually read a textbook.

His tolerance waiting for us to dredge something half memorised from a cardiology lecture exhausted, he turned to the straining face of Izzy, a hyper-earnest Australian student. He'd stopped asking her questions first, as it was pointless: she almost always had the answer. As it was, she was straining to control herself with this one – almost in physical pain holding the answer in.

With a sigh: 'Izzy, you going to put us out of our misery, then?' – his tone suggesting he was sick enough of her voice being the only response to his questions that *his* misery was now maxed out.

'Predominantly class three – but it also has some class one, two and four activity.'

The pressure valve released, the expression of a Crufts prize-winning spaniel receiving a rosette and a treat spread across her face.

'Yes,' he replied, almost imperceptibly rolling his eyes. 'Well done.'

Our Australian medical student counterparts, also visiting the hospital, clearly seemed to have missed the memo about what this elective was supposed to be about. They showed up every day, on time – and what's worse, they actually knew stuff. When there wasn't a ward round, they would be getting stuck in, speaking to patients, examining them, taking blood and generally being useful. Basically, completely dumping cold water on the idea that theirs was a 'chill' nation.

Now, as a responsible member of the medical establishment, my official message to any students on elective is to immerse yourself in this new and foreign medical system – learn as much as you can, drink in the opportunity. But also, you're away with your friends one last time before tumbling into the foundation programme meat grinder. Live a little.

The ward rounds themselves in Apia might have under-whelmed your typical Indiana Jones medic, since much of what we were seeing was disease you'd encounter at home, like bog standard heart failure and gall stones, just managed with less fuss and fewer resources.

The one exception was something we might perceive as a Victorian-era classic, but was rife there: typhoid. It seemed to take up half the paediatric ward, fevers ratcheting up by the day as worried parents looked on. The antibiotic of choice was Chloramphenicol – relegated to use in eye drops in the UK because of some rare but nasty unwanted potential side effects when taken systemically – including switching off patients' bone marrow. In Samoa, however, it was what was available – and, importantly, it worked.

The tour of the ward would often finish in the early afternoon, and being less eager than our Australian colleagues, we would head back home. At this time of day, the packs of stray dogs would still be sluggishly sunning themselves before their dusk roaming made the journey more perilous.

At the hostel, despite best intentions, we often didn't do anything constructive, of course. Many days would be spent vegetating in the heat of the main communal space. This was a wide, high-ceilinged white box, with antique wooden fans that spun lazily, regardless of the temperature. Otherwise, we cowered under the dorm-room air conditioning for some respite. Ryan, usually a ball of energy, who to this day remains unable to sit still, even as an intensive care consultant, was so idle, he completed a childhood's worth of Nintendo DS games in a week.

There were other travellers in the hostel, including a group of lads, who, unlike their medical student fellow countrymen, couldn't have been more stereotypically Australian if they'd been genetically engineered using genetic material from the cast of *Neighbours* and grown in vats of Fosters. Of the four of them, three were nearly a foot taller than me. Musclebound at a time before *Love Island* had quite had the same effect on British youth, they lounged in their inexhaustible wardrobe of 'singlets'.

The highlight of the trip for them apparently was listening to the entirety of the annual Triple J Hottest 100 radio countdown in the lounge, cheering their favourite songs with lukewarm Vailima local lager. Still, they were friendly, happy to overlook our comparative grey, British excuse for manliness.

We did head out to experience the delights of Apia, and there were bars near the harbour, many populated by sun-baked and booze-soaked expats (that word we reserve for immigrants of certain origins and hue). One disturbingly memorable conversation with a couple of leather-hided, open-shirted men (more Australians) in their fifties consisted of them tortuously and creepily comparing the art of seduction to lobster fishing. At the weekends, an ancient ferry of questionable seaworthiness would be transformed into a party liner. It chugged around the harbour playing a mix of All Bar One friendly bangers to a mix of locals, visiting students and tourists. Rum and Red Bull flowed.

Boat parties sound fun for a few seconds before you consider the practicalities – a floating raft of drunks sharing limited toilet facilities, with the captain having the final say in when you call it a night and head home. One of the Aussies, in an attention-grabbing display, took matters into his own hands one night, diving off the top deck and swimming ashore. This was met with consternation by the hosts, a talking-to from the harbour master and a promise that if anyone did anything similar, it would result in a lifetime ban for the whole group. With limited night-time entertainment options, the line was toed from then on.

* * *

I am not a golf guy. It's something I have always known instinctively I'd be terrible at, and is often played by the type of people I'd rather not spend more time around than strictly necessary (#notallgolfers – I'm sure many of you are great people). There was nothing else happening that day, however, and everyone was going – so that was enough to sway me.

The course was a heavily manicured expanse of green lawns carved into the countryside, emerging in sudden, abrupt contrast to the lush surrounding trees. It was the first and last time I have set foot on one to play. Putting any ecological concerns aside, as far as settings go, the place was beautiful, and I am happy to go out on this high. In any case, I spent the day predictably swiping and hacking hopelessly at the ball.

Seb, the palest among us and poshest among us (being the product of a notorious public school), was acutely aware of the risks posed to his alabaster skin anywhere sunnier than Putney. He had taken to applying cream with the diligence and frequency of an actor in a public safety infomercial. At the seventh hole, having topped up his coat, he squelched over to tee off. After giving a full swing with commendable follow-through, he found his hands empty. The club had glided out of his well-oiled palms, over a chain-link fence, and landed high out of sight in a dense thicket of mango trees.

'Fuck!'

'Smooth. You going to go up and get that?'

Ryan had collapsed, bent double in theatrical fits of laughter. Seb weighed up the cost of losing a golf club against the fact he hadn't climbed a tree in 15 years – and was in a country in which the provision of major trauma care could be described as 'limited'.

As he deliberated, we noticed some movement on the other side of the fence and, for the first time, voices. They were speaking excitedly and getting closer. They belonged to a group of kids – ranging from perhaps 8 to 13.

'You lose your club?'

Seb looked sheepish – the pink of his sun-afflicted face topped up with the flush of embarrassment.

'Yeah I did actually.'

'That's gonna be expensive.'

He tutted knowingly. The oldest had come forward and leaned against the fence, pressing his face up close. He wasn't wrong; golf is still a bougie business in Samoa, like most other places, and the prices for lost or damaged clubs were steep.

'You want us to help?'

'What do you mean?'

'We can get your club back.'

'Really? That would be great.'

'But you have to pay.'

'How much?'

'Forty Tala.'

He thought about this for a moment.

'Twenty.'

At this point I interjected, keen to bring to a close this scene straight out of the golden days of the Empire.

'Seb, you can't barter with a kid you're about to send up a mango tree to retrieve your golf club – just pay him!'

'Okay, half now, and half when you come back with it.'

The kid thought about this for a few seconds.

'Deal.'

With that, he walked back over to one of the other younger, and presumably more easily coerced, among the group and whispered in his ear. He quickly and obediently near-walked up the tree, as if someone had carved a staircase into the side, and was soon out of sight.

We traced his movements around the canopy by the thrashing

sounds and swaying branches. Anxiously looking on, we collectively realised how little practical medicine we knew – and how little use we would be if faced with a 'child falls from tree following colonialist golf mishap' paediatric emergency. Soon after, however, he returned holding the iron, presenting it trophy-like, chrome gleaming in the sun.

The triumph caught and spread among the group. This was the quickest money any of them had ever made. Seb begrudgingly handed over the rest of the money, and the crowd left, made giddy by the spoils.

Seb spent the remainder of the holes sulking, fully aware that this cloak of ridicule, the green jacket of shame, would be worn for the remainder of the day, perhaps the week, or even the rest of his life.

This was a low point – the interaction shattering any pretence there may have been about the tradition we were part of. Namely, that rather than really helping, we were foreign tourists, spending the day on the other side of the fence in a club most locals couldn't access – only interacting with them when we needed something.

* * *

It wouldn't be international adventure travel without someone getting sick or injured – although, as I say, for a tropical island, Samoa hosts a surprising lack of wildlife and microbes out to kill you. What can't be avoided wherever you are, however, is good old-fashioned gastroenteritis. And when it comes to a band of young men together in a room, with 'basic' washing facilities – if one of you gets it, all of you get it.

The dorms were in a separate two-storey concrete block. Our group had been divided – with four in one room, and three in the other. Amid the horse-trading for beds, I ended up with what felt like a favourable lot, namely fewer roommates – just Kyron and Ryan.

The first gurglings sounded in the larger group – and soon everyone in that room progressed from 'feeling a little delicate' to porcelain-shatteringly unwell. They were quarantined – left to fester in a soup of tropical sweat and shaky bowels. I'm thankful to this day I wasn't in there, and by some miracle our room remained unscathed.

No one was sure where they could have caught it – it's not like we were eating anything too adventurous most days. The closest we had to street food was the roti kiosk at the hospital. Otherwise, a lot of the meals we prepared in the tiny hostel kitchen for ourselves came out of a packet.

We were reliant on the supermarket, which often meant ramen noodles and meat, the processed kind – because that's what was affordable. This was exacerbated by unfamiliarity with the local vegetables, like the staple tarot – which, honestly, I'd have no idea what to do with even if you gave it to me with detailed instructions and a how-to video. Fancy anything imported, like lettuce on the other hand, and we'd have had to save up, because at least where we were, it cost almost as much as a steak.

The one thing that likely saved us from crippling constipation (other than the aforementioned outbreak) was the array of fruit from the hostel's grounds laid out at breakfast, which would have put the spread at the finest Dubai hotels to shame. The table heaved with spine-covered lychees, papaya and squat miniature bananas.

Fruit aside, the imbalance in our diets may not be that surprising. As visitors we didn't have daily access to the produce many families grow on their land. Every now and then we would get a glimpse, a bite of traditional Samoan cuisine, whenever staff at the hospital would prepare a communal lunch, or we were invited to an event at a nearby village. Then we had *palusami* (tarot leaves in coconut milk) and *oka* (raw marinated fish) – both dishes you could imagine some influencer gushing over as if they have just 'discovered' the next big thing.

But the far-reaching grip of globalised trade also means Samoan diets are shifting, to include more imported meat, vegetable oil and those oh-so-nutritious and delicious instant noodles. It would be rich for me, off the back of a jaunt to the other side of the world, to return warning of the dangers of polluting indigenous cultures with our Western poison, but on the hospital ward we met a 35-year-old man with end-stage kidney disease due to diabetes, and the number of Samoans needing dialysis as a result of metabolic syndrome-related disease has skyrocketed since the beginning of the century.

Alongside these effects of access to apparently irresistible Western culinary offerings, Samoa's strategic location in the South Pacific means someone bigger will always be interested in having their say locally. Two hundred and twenty kilometres to the east, a whole crop of islands is glaringly named 'American Samoa' – for historical . . . reasons. On a smaller scale, the hospital in Apia boasted a new CT scanner which had been benevolently donated by the Chinese government, with, I'm certain, absolutely no ulterior motives or strings attached. Of course, Samoa was under British colonial administration until 1962, so we are hardly in a position to talk.

With invasive cultures, it's impossible to predict which cultural snares will take hold. A visit in 2019 from famous vaccine 'sceptic' (to put it mildly) Robert F. Kennedy Junior is viewed by many as fuelling a measles outbreak in the country. More innocuously, on a trip to a village out of town, as well as the prized marinated fish, we were gifted a CD recorded by a local band. For reasons none of us could quite grasp, but that the locals felt were self-evident, and therefore didn't need explaining, the album was dedicated to Princess Diana. Her presence clearly endures there almost as much as on the covers of UK tabloid media.

Other than Lady Di and Christianity, which is almost ubiquitous across the two islands that make up Samoa, the import that has embedded itself most firmly was summed up by one phrase:

'Go da Manu!'

The slogan, in support of the Samoan rugby team, was everywhere – painted on the side of trucks, on the radio and on the lips of the people of Apia.

During our stay, Samoa were competing in the Rugby Sevens World Series, close to home in Wellington New Zealand. It's kind of a big deal. For a country of only 200,000 people, like many other Pacific islands, Samoa can seem like a rugby player factory – a production line churning out high-speed human wrecking balls. Like Jamaica with sprinting, you could have many a problematic debate regarding genetics vs environment, straying quickly into the swamp of race science. Whatever the reason, the national team were pretty good.

On game days, things ground to a standstill. The streets seemed deserted of cars, and every bar and local shop hosted an excited throng gathered around a small blaring TV. Casualties included teams from Japan, Scotland and Canada – the team reached the semi-finals, only losing out to their larger Fijian cousins. This might have been for the best; had they won the whole thing I'm not convinced we would have survived the ensuing celebrations.

* * *

In the latter weeks of our time in Apia, we settled into the rhythms of the hospital, becoming less work-shy and even knowing the answers to some questions. We still weren't on a par with our Antipodean counterparts when it came to keenness – but really, no one needed that. I continued alternating between the adult medical and paediatrics wards, while Ryan and Tommy honed their (supervised) long needle skills with the anaesthetists, as they delivered spinal anaesthetics.

On our final night, and despite the looming early wake-up call, there was a party at the hostel. Pops, the owner of said hostel, and a man who initially matched Dr Keil in his gruffness, but had gradually warmed during our stay, gathered the seven of us in a circle to offer an interruption to the bottles of Vai Lima.

He had a bowl of Kava, or 'Ava – a drink found across Polynesia, with particular ritual significance in Samoa. We took turns drinking the thin, chocolate milk-coloured liquid, unsure what to expect, both in terms of taste and purported psychoactive effects. The flavour I can best describe as neutral – the consensus seems to be Kava is 'earthy', but thankfully it hasn't left me with some deep, unforgettable sense memory, so it can't have been that bad (which is more than can be said for many spirits). The effects, between the alcohol and heightened emotion of moving on, are hard to separate – but in combination, the recollection is of warm nostalgia.

I'm not sure what we went through would qualify as a by-the-book Kava ceremony, and there are always the optics of foreigners indulging tokenistically in local traditions, but nevertheless, it was an expression of hospitality and friendship that remains with me.

With any trip like this, it would be delusional to believe you've had anything more than an outsider's glimpse of a country. Even staying somewhere for weeks on end, you are part of a transient, migrating community and can't make any sensible claim to really understand the culture. It's also inevitable that, in reporting, you risk stumbling into the outdated history of travellers reporting back on their experience of the 'exotic'.

Ultimately, this sort of travel is valuable to medics – and particularly once trained, we can hopefully do some good in the places we go. But if you want to know what the people in these places think of us showing up, you'd have to ask them. And if you want to know about Samoan and islander culture, their lives and the issues they face, seek out their work. Outside of Samoa, in places like New Zealand the contribution of writers and other artists of Samoan heritage is increasingly being recognised, but it is still early days. In the UK, as a *MasterChef* devotee, we have Monica Galetti, and then there is, of course, global megastar Dwayne 'the Rock' Johnson.

CHAPTER 14

Marches on Its Stomach

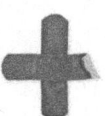

PEOPLE PUT UP signs, they clapped for carers – but the one thing that has actually made us feel appreciated is the food. After the first delivery, it has arrived every day without fail: plastic Tupperware filled with gratitude measured by the forkful. Restaurants, deprived of customers, have emptied their walk-in freezers into the hospital.

Soon after a premium food delivery drops, a network of spies is alerted and the word goes out over WhatsApp. As long as I'm not doing something truly time-sensitive or life-saving, it's a cue to excuse myself and slink off to the staff room in the emergency department.

Everything that's been given is gratefully received – the nearby Sikh temple have essentially kept me alive with their donations. At this point in the pandemic, deep brown, glistening dhal is probably creeping through my veins. But today's crate is paying out the jackpot: sushi rolls. They will be gone in minutes, and I have no intention of missing out, my selflessness only going so far. Sure, there may be someone more deserving, someone who has worked harder today, but on this occasion, I just don't care. I compose a message to Shivani, the geriatrics registrar also attached to Dr Sharp's ward, with the news and get an immediate response.

'How do you always get down there so quickly? Is there anything good left?'

As well as the heads up, I had the added benefit that I was already working in the ED – proximity to the food being one of the few perks.

'Maybe, if you're quick . . .'

Shivani has never been lucky – this is well documented. Relatives making impossible demands? Check. Half her team members calling in sick at once and leaving her looking after 20 patients by herself? Check. Said patients inexplicably spontaneously combusting? Give it time – but, undoubtedly, check.

This is her first registrar job, ST3 – arguably the most daunting step up in a junior doctor's career, having to manage others, suddenly supposed to *really* know things. On call, other teams will ask you to come and review their patients, dole out your learned pearls of wisdom. I struggle to believe it, but despite being far more diligent and hardworking, she seems to think I have useful advice to give her on handling this change – my meagre added experience suddenly counting for something.

On the days when there isn't a consultant ward round, as the SpR, you're the boss – deciding who's doing what, who's seeing who and in what order. If it reaches lunchtime with only half the ward seen, it's on you.

It is a sad truth that almost everything delicious is something your well-meaning healthcare provider will tell you off for eating. We know this, but as the biscuits and chocolates adorning any self-respecting hospital workstation will attest, we are often no better. When it comes to dessert, I have the self-restraint of a sweet-toothed five-year-old actively courting type-2 diabetes.

When we tell patients what not to eat during a 15-minute consultation, we can be taking away much more than just a snack and a few percentage points of risk. With food, we ask them to give up their most visceral of memories, ones reawakened and sublimed into the air as the flame touches the pan, onions becoming caramel, garlic roasting in hot fat.

A pie isn't just crust, gravy and saturated fat – within the pastry is held the reminiscence of football on a Saturday, conjured in the pitch-green liquor. Curry goat isn't just an indulgence spiked with your daily recommended salt allowance, but rather the past bubbles from beneath the surface – like the time when my grandad arranged catering for my aunt's wedding, and a goat arrived alive, kicking and intent on eating the entire garden. My grandmother's roses, my grandfather's nerves and the goat all never recovered. Not only being able to cope with the spice, and the rich earthy funk of the meat, but actually enjoying it was a mark of pride for my seven-year-old self – signifying a mature, adventurous spirit, but also belonging. Very few people have Proustian, transportive experiences over steamed broccoli.

This is the point where a slow-motion, ultra HD shot documents the expert dicing of a shallot, before it is purposefully tossed into the sizzling pool of oil and toasted spices – all while the narration breathily and reverentially speaks to the spiritual and cultural importance of cooking dinner. What can I say? When it comes to the po-faced exaltation of getting dinner ready, so characteristic of the earnest Netflix cooking shows, I'm all in.

People who like the good things in life, that are so bad for us, are often the most fun to be around. As a doctor working in rheumatology I shouldn't say this, but I have yet to meet the patient with poorly controlled gout, who really should cut down on the red meat and wine, who isn't a bit of a laugh. They are the ones I'd ask for restaurant recommendations – even though they're doing their health no favours.

A dish, a cooking tradition so charged with history, subtext and a seasoning of undeserving shame that I almost daren't bring it up, is fried chicken. There is reluctance to admit that among the crowning achievements of humanity (culinary or otherwise) has been the introduction of chicken to batter, followed swiftly by a shotgun marriage in a cathedral of oil. It is denigrated as unsophisticated, in no small part due to the association with the marginalised – namely black people, especially poor black people.

In the form we know it, fried chicken emerged as a staple of cooking from the Southern US states. The origins are unclear – some have connected it to spiced and fried recipes from Western Africa, areas many enslaved people and their descendants trace their ancestry to. It has been pointed out, however, that battering and deep-frying it in fat also likely bares the influence of Scottish traditions. My mother will punch the air triumphantly if this is ever proved to be true (but I'm not about to risk the level of controversy fully endorsing this theory would bring). Regardless of the provenance of that first kernel of an idea, what we recognise today undoubtedly comes from the kitchens on plantations, perfected and cooked by stolen people.

There is very little, if anything, that tastes better – it's as if we all just needed permission to acknowledge it, and it is happening. As with so many things, white hipster culture has taken this long-shunned, complex-historied black staple, repackaged it and sold it back to the gullible masses at triple the price. These places will never replace the chicken shop, however, the ultra-bright high street focal points that serve as restaurants-come-meeting points. They become geographic signifiers – south Londoners showing an often-irrational level of Morley's devotion.

But whatever form it comes in, I love it – health consequences, social connotations be damned. It was often fried, rather than jerk, chicken that my grandmother cooked on the rare occasions our whole family managed to get together when we were young. Besides, almost every culture has their version, or something close. However, European versions are freed from the burden of stigma – the worst someone will say about you serving a chicken Kyiv is that it's a little retro.

Many of my colleagues will read this aghast and think what I've said is irresponsible. I am under no illusions that fried chicken is doing anything good for my life expectancy. Like Nas said:

'Fried chicken, fly vixen

Give me heart disease, but need you in my kitchen.'

I assure you I'm not minimising the importance of eating well and exercising in the name of health and reducing the risk of chronic disease. It isn't controversial to suggest everyone should be aiming to max out on the fresh fruit and vegetables, and minimise sugar and ultra-processed food (although this can be frustratingly difficult to define). It's just our current approach, one that ignores the wider cultural and emotional context of food, is delusional. This is evidenced when you look at the figures. It clearly isn't working.

This is before considering that a lot of the worst food for us is cheap, with the inevitable consequence that many of the poorest will be pushed towards unhealthy choices. Telling a person with limited funds to fill up a hessian sack with artisanal produce at whole foods, or a farmers' market, over a cheaper and less time-intense processed meal is naive.

We are still in the habit of demonising people for their health, and for their physical response to food. Fatness is framed as a failing, rather than an interaction between their genetics and the environment – and, in turn, we blame the individual. It must be due to some personal weakness, a choice being made. We ignore the truth that the effects of a given calorific intake, range of foods and amount of exercise will have a different impact on different individuals, governed by their physiology. Pretty much everyone seems happy to accept that as we age, we're likely to pile on a few, to 'let ourselves go', thanks to our metabolism. The idea that we might all be starting from a different point, however, with some of us prone to getting fatter at any age, apparently seems too far-fetched to entertain.

A direction of travel that will no doubt trigger the dreaded accusation of 'wokery' from more senior voices, there is a trend towards checking patients are actually on board with the treatments we're proposing. Patient involvement is a vital part of the planning, funding and ethics approval of any modern clinical study. If you ask many people labelled as 'fat' or 'obese', they'll tell you they feel stigmatised by a lot of what healthcare professionals say and do in the name of helping them shed weight.

This might arguably be less of an issue if the weight-loss inter-ventions worked for a majority of patients, but a lot of our historic and current approaches seem to be close to pissing in the wind. Even the most intensive calorie-restricted diet data, trumpeted as a success, has shown what I would argue are less than landscape-shifting results. Telling someone to live on a mainly liquid diet indefinitely, for a 5 per cent chance of keeping the weight off after five years, is a pitch even the most psychotically overconfident *Apprentice* candidate wouldn't back themselves to make.

Of course, the weight-loss injections Wegovy and Mounjaro,

beloved of the red carpet (that temple to health), are being touted as miracle cures to all that I have described, and potentially much else besides. The outcomes of their long-term use for this indication remain to be seen, however. There is also not the infrastructure or funding to dole them out like the forbidden smarties they're designed to stop you craving.

For now, we are left making a hell of a lot of people feeling terrible, in the hope of helping a very small number. I'm not advocating nihilism, but rather a change of approach, one where people are empowered, both financially and through education, to make healthier choices.

* * *

'I'm on my way, is there anything good left?'

The message lets me know Shivani has finally managed to escape, having finished what was looking like a never-ending round.

The brief interval between the notification and her walking in suggests she jogged down from the ward, dodging dawdlers and trolleys in the corridors. As she approaches the table, her shoulders are already slumped in defeat, and she peers inside the box. Unexpectedly, miraculously even, the seagulls in scrubs and stethoscopes have been slow, and she plucks out a sushi roll.

'You know I'm probably going to get hit by a car on the way home to balance this out, don't you?'

'Oh, obviously – if anyone could get run over when the streets of London are deserted, it's you.'

The staff room at lunch time is where hospital gossip finds oxygen – ironically today the topic is the alarms ringing throughout the halls, apparently a warning we're dangerously close to running out, thanks to the number of patients having their breathing supported by CPAP machines.

It's also where you really get to meet the people you work with, get to look into their lives. In less well-catered times, it could be the sad meal deal betraying the home life of the FY1 – who is too time-poor to prepare a lunch, and between student loans, rent and exam fees, too cash-strapped to swallow the price of something warm but disappointing from the canteen. Or it could be the ward sister's jollof rice, my hunger dialled up by every degree it warms in the microwave.

And then there is the Filipino ED nurses' lunch club – an event unto itself. Unloaded like precious cargo smuggled into the hospital, the members watch over it expectantly – as I look on with confusion, quickly giving way to envy when someone explains they do this every Friday. Pork, rice and lumpia for lunch – no one ever told me this was an option. It feels like they've found some cheat code.

The array of meals on display is a reminder of the one thing that even the staunchest xenophobe would struggle to deny: immigration makes food better. It always has. Even in times of conquest, the sword is accompanied by the spatula. Unfortunately, we have Portuguese colonialism to thank for the introduction of chilli to India – although to be fair, afterwards, the people of the subcontinent really did run with it and make it their own – and down the line, we get our 'national dish': a curry. I have never met a skinhead that doesn't love a curry. Pretty quickly things change from 'get out of my country' to 'get in my mouth'.

A penchant for a plant-based diet has become associated with a certain strand of the white middle class – and raw veganism in particular is the domain of the fad-susceptible, yoga-wear-sporting influencer. But others have been doing it for years; the more devout Rastafarians subscribe to an Ital diet – vegan, as unprocessed food as possible, and often raw. And of course the

Indian subcontinent is host to many vegetarian and vegan food cultures, the 'borrowed' recipes from which are probably keeping the majority of plant-based westerners alive.

It would be too easy, and also unfair, to pretend all traditional British food (whatever that truly is) is bland, stodgy and not worth giving much thought to. Places like St John, in revisiting these dishes, have made that position untenable. Self-professed 'foodies', simultaneously easily persuaded and in the know, pay handsomely for kidneys and bone marrow on toast. But without immigration, I can be certain I'd look forward to eating out much less.

* * *

As I have already alluded to, in some ways, being a doctor is a lot like being a chef, while in others, they couldn't be further apart. The hours are long, you're on your feet for much of the time, often without a toilet break, and you cater to a public that can unpredictably veer wildly from adulation and gratitude to ominous demands to speak with the manager. We both experience the nervous simmer in the build-up to being slammed on a Saturday night – knowing we will pay for the moment's breath taken during the relative calm of the morning later on, when we are 'in the shit'. And of course you're hopefully always washing your hands.

Having spent some time around chefs growing up (one of my best friends dropped out of sixth form and joined a kitchen, like running away to the circus), however I also know how we are different. From what I have heard from him, everything that has become cliche after exposés such as Anthony Bourdain's memoir *Kitchen Confidential* seems to have more than a grain of truth – many brigades being full of oddballs and dropouts who couldn't function in any sane, HR-regulated environment. As a result, they're willing to work punishing hours, for a salary that makes no sense (on second thought, conditions FY1s can relate to).

I have never set foot in a professional kitchen for more than a few minutes – but I have certainly seen what they get up to outside. Drinks at the bar, or on the kerb out by the service entrance in summer, escalate until half the kitchen wakes up in the manager's flat above the restaurant, bodies and gossip strewn everywhere. The next day's shift and the accompanying mountain of prep form the rapidly approaching concrete reality check, as they fall back to earth from last night's high.

On the other hand, many chefs *do* also seem to care as much about doing the job well as many of my colleagues, more even. They'll unironically and earnestly tell you of the extra hours of their own time spent perfecting a parfait, in the hope of getting it on the menu – as if the producers of *MasterChef: The Professionals* are secretly filming from behind a plant pot. They sound like trainee surgeons, coming in on one of their rare days off to practise their skills in theatre (and, it goes without saying, suck up to an influential consultant).

Chefs have had to deal with the megalomaniacal whims and tempers of their bosses – something all junior doctors will recognise. Although reform is happening in both instances, work often carries the ever-present threat of ritual public humiliation and punishment, in the case of chefs even physical. I have seen first-hand footage of an unfortunate commis, who after one fuck-up too many was forced to endure the kitchen's go-to disciplinary procedure – arms outstretched to the side, Passion of the Christ-style, holding heavy cast-iron pans, as he was dangled in front of the hottest burner on the stove, gently roasting like some carcass on a spit.

One well-known TV chef has the reputation of having settled

kitchen scores in the most primitive way imaginable back in the day. Offenders would be invited into the meat freezer and offered out for some bare-knuckle discipline – tenderised into promising the veal is never overcooked again. Presumably the need to keep face (and one's job) was enough to compel chefs to treat boxing with the boss as a normal part of their daily routine. I am only aware of one disagreement in any of the hospitals I have worked in coming to blows – with an intensivist chinning a surgeon on the ward, euphemistically labelled as a 'heated discussion' in the GMC report on the incident.

Some stars can lose sight of the reason they cook in the first place – instead serving up a procession of fellow-chef-pleasing artworks, concepts. Assisted by brigades numbering in the dozens, they'd sooner shut up shop than run a service without their micro-herb tweezering guy. There can be a tacit contempt for those working more provincially, with fewer resources, but giving the customer what they want and need.

Some ivory-tower medics come close to the same self-indulgent myopia. By the time you are practising a sub-speciality of a sub-speciality, at a hospital attached to one of this country's finest higher learning institutions, with a well-staffed team of eager research fellows keen to impress you, suddenly doing 'good medicine', and by extension looking down on the work of others, becomes surprisingly easy. This may be great for the desperate and grateful patient in front of you, overjoyed that you have finally diagnosed their 'whatthefuckisititis'. Just remember you had time and help that aren't available to humble journeymen cranking out dinners (diagnoses) at the neighbourhood bistro (district general hospital).

Food is the main area I'll admit to embracing extravagance. I don't care about cars, I sometimes have to remind myself to buy clothes to avoid looking destitute – but I do care about where and what I eat. If I'm travelling, the first thing that's looked up is where to have dinner, and the menu. That said, cost of living, coupled with the realities of having a small child, mean that now most culinary indulgence is confined to the home. I'm not playing around with gels and I don't have a stash of liquid nitrogen, but I did spend about as much on my barbecue as I did on my first car (although said vehicle *was* that barely held-together soapbox cart of a Corsa).

Food is how I connect with my friends, it's how I show people I care – and it really matters. When company, food and drink align, for me they are the closest moments come to some transcendent ideal. For better or worse, how well I pull off the cooking at these times affects my mood. It's far from healthy, but if I'm cooking and it goes wrong, ruining a meal feels like making a mistake at work.

What we eat can all too often be a reminder of class and culture, in a Britain still far too obsessed with such things. Almost foreshadowing the current middle-class no sugar movement, growing up, our parents restricted our access to the corner shop, no matter how much we protested. They would counter that the '10p mix' we were allowed on a Saturday was more than enough. Other kids were allowed to wander daily into this emporium of instant gratification, sat on the corner of the school run thoroughfare like a cavity-toothed crocodile on the edge of a watering hole.

But nor were we from the sort of family who spend the average daily wage on artisanal olive oils and jars of artichokes and sun-dried tomatoes without thinking. This was before the turn-of-the-century New Labour hummus revolution – such things were still the preserve of those that, despite leaning left, when push came to shove still sent their kids to private school and holidayed in the south of France.

Regardless of how anglicised my dad may seem to some with a narrow understanding, his cooking was often still Jamaican. His Saturday afternoon staple when looking after us was saltfish fritters, and most meals he cooked came with a side of plantain, no matter how indifferent my brother and I were to its charms – the cultural traitors we are.

Even today, admitting to not liking plantain as a child feels like risking ostracism. One now internationally famous black UK comedian once swore me to secrecy, when at a party they admitted that they too weren't the biggest fan of it. I am, however, proud to say that after a long struggle, the maturation of my palate, and some soul-searching, I *do* like plantain, as long as it's not too sweet.

Given food is this door to culture, to a soul even, I'm a sucker for beautifully shot food travel docs, where the host visits far-flung corners of the globe, eating their way to discovery. They'll sit down with a diverse range of storied individuals for a meal, while hearing about their lives – before inevitably coming to the satisfying realisation over a plate of hummus made to a secret family recipe, barbecued meat or noodle soup, that we're all more similar than we are different, and food is what brings people together, how we communicate our cultures.

I'm not so naive or blinkered, however, to ignore the fact that many of these destinations where we have been shown such idylls have descended back into conflict and despair following these visits. But at the same time, my optimism persists that any reconciliation and progress is going to involve food – much like the first thing many of us did as soon as we were allowed, when COVID restrictions lifted, was to meet and welcome our friends into our homes to eat, eager as we were to reclaim the connection that we had been denied.

Not every meal can be a savoured bonding, and medicine has ruined my table manners. The dread of the bleep means I now eat lunch like I'm worried someone is about to slap it out of my hand and take the plate – hunched over and shovelling at speed. Near-constant interruptions and abruptly curtailed breaks teach you this.

Much like now. In the time it has taken to stuff half a roll into her face, Shivani has been bleeped twice. Both times she stopped to answer; the query was something pretty inane that could have waited, but there's no way of telling until you pick up the phone. The third bleep sounded more like a real wolf, however, and that was that, break over. With a heavy sigh, she packed up her lunch and trudged back upstairs.

Still, having the opportunity to sit together, even briefly, in whatever numbers and at whatever distance was permitted at the time, was a small piece of normality that made the whole experience that bit more bearable.

CHAPTER 15

I Can't Breathe

BY MAY 2020, days of the week in the hospital had ceased to have much meaning. Medical teams worked in rolling patterns that dotted the calendar with responsibilities of greater and lesser levels of intensity. On 25 May, a Monday, I had arrived at my downtime, a weekday 'weekend' – having been the HDU SpR for the previous three days: twelve-hour shifts of donning and doffing a PPE space suit in the hope of keeping the unfortunate breathing.

Out of sync, I waited each day for Louise, who was now a GP trainee, to get back from the surgery. Like the rest of her primary-care colleagues, she had been forced to add the novel uncertainties of phone consultations to the high-risk lottery of general practice – the worry being that in keeping a vulnerable patient out of the surgery, avoiding infection, you miss the subtle signs of something really wrong.

Before this sounds too much like self-pity, recuperation took place under much more pleasant circumstances than others were experiencing. We had a garden, so can look back on the first lockdown with something verging on nostalgia – for the peace of days off that were sun-drenched and motionless. We weren't hemmed into a cramped flat, allowed only brief, overpoliced forays into the air outside. We weren't subject to the rising suffocation experienced by communities who were growing tired of feeling the brunt of ills, both viral and societal.

Where you get your news from, the conversations you're plugged into, matters – the pandemic most certainly showed us this. And when it came to the murder of George Floyd, all I can do is admit that I missed it, what was really important, the reality of the situation, even though all the details were there.

I remember seeing the story that Monday after it happened, information trickling out of the narrow stream from which I reflexively draw most news. Sitting outside, I read that another black American had died at the hands of the police. I remember feeling what, at this point, had become my default pessimism. That it would change nothing – and that his name would be added to those of Philando Castile, Breonna Taylor and so many others.

I missed the point, that this was a modern-day lynching caught on camera, captured in horrifying detail – all 8 minutes and 46 seconds of callous homicidal pressure applied to a man's neck, the full weight of a perpetrator who felt his status as the law made him invincible. This time around, however, things were different – it wouldn't just be a committed minority speaking out, but a whole section of society, whose lives, it had been made clear by a pandemic, by the actions of the police, didn't matter to those with power, on account of their blackness.

These embers found oxygen online – and by the following Saturday, the growing number of posts had spilled out into action. Separated by thousands of miles, but united in recognition and frustration, there was a weekend of response, both online and on the UK streets.

* * *

Watching Interventional Radiology through the glass is, at turns, both remarkable and dull. The operator is attempting life-saving miracles in the patient's circulatory system, fishing out a clot, sealing a bleeding aneurysm, or propping open an artery with the end of a wire, like a glorified coat hanger hooking a set of keys through the letterbox – only stealing back life, rather than the Audi from the driveway.

What this amounts to visually, however, is staring at the back of a hyper-focused, hunched figure. They roll the wire between thumb and forefinger like Rizla papers, bending and traversing some corner, and then delicately feeding in more steel.

The payoff for the spectator comes in the position check – the catheter is injected, flooding the arachnid limbs of the vessel with iodine. The dye branches out across the fluoroscopy screen, hopefully confirming the culprit has been reached.

Today, this was taking longer than usual. To be fair to the radiologist, we had lumbered them with a real shitter of a case. Literally. Somewhere in this woman's guts, she had sprung a leak, and blood is a highly effective, highly unpleasant laxative. Melaena, the treacle-black results of bleeding high up the gastrointestinal tract, makes the toilet bowl look like an oil spill, while bleeding from lower down progresses from deep crimson to bright scarlet. The emergency endoscopy of the top end, normally the first port of call, hadn't shown much, so the problem had to be beyond the reach of the scope.

A CT mapping the blood supply to the abdomen had revealed the source, a deceptively small artery supplying the bowel was hosing into the passage. With the leak identified, the next mountain was finding someone to fix it. In her eighties, the patient was frail by surgical standards, and the combination of an emergency anaesthetic and the controlled stabbing of an operation might have been enough to finish her off.

Fortunately, she had the good sense to pitch up to a hospital with a wire-fiddler happy to take on the task – by no means a guarantee. Their skill set comes with the dual benefit of only needing to punch a comparatively small hole in the groin to get at the problem, and keeping you awake while doing so, minimising anaesthetic risk.

With her in the radiologist's hands, I was there just in case – on standby nearby should the bleeding gather pace and destabilise things, or a stray flick of the steel shear the vessel and open up a second front. In that scenario, it would be my job to coordinate any resuscitation attempts and pump blood and fluid back in, hopefully faster than it was rushing out.

Nothing of the sort looked like happening, leaving me with idle thumbs outside, in the viewing gallery.

I don't enjoy social media. This isn't a value judgement, just a reaction to the way using it feels. I try to stay off it, but I'm not immune to passively lurking and reading from time to time. With little to see from the procedure, like any member of my addled generation, the reflex in this scenario was to turn to my phone.

I don't let Twitter nudge me out of real life with a needy vibrational tug for every notification, but there was still the red dot over the app symbol on the home screen, a siren call to open up and see what new mention was there to validate my importance. Looking at the updates, I felt the blood leave my face faster than the patient on the table. My contribution to the conversation surrounding the most emotional, most contentious of events in the world outside had been received like a plate of foie gras at a PETA meeting.

Earlier, I had seen a tweet by Imani, a friend from south-east London, drawn from a large group who spent our twenties staying out past any civilised bedtime at friends' basement club nights. She admonished those who had stayed silent, and those who had only spoken up belatedly, after being called out. The thought of being among them had weighed shamefully.

'Suddenly got something to say . . . Trying to jump on this train when it's already gone and left the station.'

Some level of guilt, whether realised or not, can make words feel like they are spoken directly to you. I had hastily composed what I was convinced would be a concise mea culpa, but unwisely tempered with self-justification, a request not to read too much into my silence – and added it to the thread.

'Tbh this could be me, but that's down to my lack of interaction with Twitter.'

If you're confused, you're not alone – reading it back now, even setting aside the shirking of responsibility, it's hard to know if the sentence even makes complete sense. It certainly doesn't say exactly what I intended it to – that I hadn't posted anything because I barely use Twitter rather than because I didn't care.

In any case, predictably, this proved unwise, unnecessarily peering above the parapet and strolling gormlessly into the middle of a digital firefight. The responses from all sides were swift, to the point, and unforgiving – landing as I stood waiting for the radiologist to finish.

Before the absolute calamity of the interaction could sink in too deeply, it was time to return to the emergency at hand. Fortunately, the bleeder had been faring a lot better than I had. The radiologist was reaching the final turn, and would soon seal off a small branch, hopefully stemming the flow. I'd be collecting the patient to be wheeled gingerly back to the ward, her fragility so great that any corner taken too fast might shatter her completely.

* * *

To say there are unresolved issues between the police and black communities in the UK would be an understatement – on a par with saying hip-hop fans were disappointed to hear Andre 3000's long-awaited 2023 project was going to be a flute album. The visibility may be different from when things were at their worst in the 1970s and 80s, but there is still a long way to go.

Memories of the Stockwell Six and Oval Four – and corrupt officers like Derek Ridgewell, who targeted young black men, framing them for robbery – will last many lifetimes. As will the treatment of the Lawrence family by the Metropolitan Police following their son's murder. When policing by consent is so degraded, and officers act to victimise and punish according to race, stealing life from the innocent, this has to be resisted.

The video of black athletes Bianca Williams and Ricardo Dos Santos being stopped and searched in July 2020 – pulled from their car and handcuffed while their three-month-old son was in the back seat, was a reminder that we may not have come as far as we think. The Team GB sprinter and her partner were pulled over and searched for drugs and weapons – apparently the only grounds for suspicion was being black in a Mercedes.

The officers claimed they smelled cannabis – an excuse countless among us have heard . . . It is a pretext that continues to be used by officers, to stop black people in particular, at will. The most ludicrous use of this excuse that springs to mind was Mani Arthur in 2019. Mr Arthur, the founder of the Black Cyclists' Network, was stopped and searched by police while riding in traffic. The officer accused him of smelling of cannabis – apparently the keenest nostrils on the force was trained to smell weed at a distance, over the smell of exhaust fumes, emanating from a man who clearly wasn't smoking, because he was *cycling*. It goes without saying that they didn't find anything.

Between March 2019 and 2020, black people were 8.9 times more likely to be stopped and searched than their white counterparts. Figures have varied by year, but at their most extreme, in England and Wales, in 2017–2018 they were 40 times more likely under certain circumstances. Hopefully none except the most diehard of bigots would suggest one ethnic group is intrinsically 40 times more likely to be committing a crime than another.

Being criminalised simply for existing in a public space, by one of the most visible manifestations of the state, is alienating. It is a reminder that the establishment, and the tools that exist to uphold it, work for some citizens, and against others. My brother and I were given the same talk by our father as most other young black men in this country: don't give the police any excuse, and don't trust them not to be racist.

This excess in policing is not harmless, not just an inconvenience. There is of course the lifetime impact of being arrested and charged with a crime. But more seriously, the reality is that the lives of black people detained by the police can be placed in danger. They are over-represented in statistics of deaths following police contact, making up 19.5 per cent of deaths in police custody compared to 3 per cent of the population.

Racism is like a variable gravity, a force that is selective as to who is held down, and by how much – and this is manifest in policing. So, all of this, and vastly more besides, was the landscape, the scorched scrubland waiting to be set alight by that video.

* * *

The first time I was stopped and searched was suitably on brand. I was picked out from an otherwise all-white group because of my race and appearance. Aged 15, I was frisked while still legally a child (admittedly older than many others when it first happens to them), without being made fully aware of my rights. But at the same time, it was on suspicion of the lamest crime imaginable.

I was at one of the 2003 Stop the Iraq War protests, an event that, though it attracted all-comers, at times looked like Carnival sponsored by Planet Organic. It happened towards the end of the day, when purposeful marching had given way to aimless milling around, but with an energy that had not yet fully dissipated. There were no more speeches to be given, the main focal points now being a few mobile speakers blaring out reggae and rave classics.

I remember the officer's face appearing in front of mine, accompanied by the realisation that despite not having perceptibly moved, I was now somehow isolated from my friends.

Less anxious than I should have been, I retained the false reassurance of someone who has done nothing wrong, and believes this fact will be more than sufficient to disentangle them from what is clearly a misunderstanding.

'We know what you've been doing.'

I stared back at him blankly – mainly out of confusion.

He continued. 'We've seen you – you've been . . . throwing apples.'

I remained silent for a moment.

'I . . . wasn't . . .'

'Don't try and deny it – we have you on camera.'

It's a strange feeling realising that one of two things must be true: either a police officer is lying, or you have a doppelganger wandering the streets of London, committing twee crimes.

'You *were* throwing apples.'

I could never have seen this coming. Apparently, I fit the description, real or imagined, of someone delinquent enough to commit acts of violence against the public and servants of the crown – but with only as deadly a weapon as an underripe Granny Smith.

He had the smug face typical of the type of loser who goes in for petty rule enforcement, when they feel they have someone bang to rights.

'Because we have reason to believe you were throwing them, and endangering the public, I'm now going to search you.'

And with that, in full view of all and sundry, and without a responsible adult present, I was frisked – in the hope they would find on my person . . . some dangerous fruit.

Being a (relatively) typical teenager, funnily enough I hadn't filled my pockets with healthy snacks, so the officer and his sidekicks didn't find what they were looking for. Frustrated, but undeterred, they changed tack. The lightbulb moment had struck: why not revert to that aforementioned stock pretext for violating civil liberties, old reliable, the one that serves them so well?

'You smell of cannabis.'

We were at a Stop the War protest – *everything* smelled of weed. Unluckily for them, I was probably one of the few exceptions. I have no moral qualms, but I am a naturally anxious person – I don't need weed adding to that. A dry mouth, racing heart and red eyes aren't my idea of a relaxing time. Also, I have asthma. As the search continued, his enthusiasm was replaced by disappointment.

'Smoked all your weed, have you?' – this exasperated last-ditch question apparently some attempt at a Jedi mind trick, designed to baffle me into suddenly confessing my crimes.

'I wasn't smoking weed,' I defiantly, if sullenly reiterated.

Finally accepting defeat, they warned me I had better behave in future – and like that it was over. They sank back into the currents of diehards and revellers that were still rolling around the square.

* * *

'Bro, I can see what you were trying to say there – but it doesn't come across.'

The catastrophe on Twitter had been almost all I had thought about the past few days, agonising over it. I had managed to make a man's murder on the other side of the world into my own personal tragedy. The intensity undoubtedly had a lot to do with the feeling of ostracism at this critical time, like confirmation of something I had often felt, like permission and acceptance being revoked.

In my desperation, I had turned to outside counsel. Leon brought the multiple benefits of being a mutual friend who is also wise, and importantly, one of the most unreasonably nice guys you'll ever meet.

Looking over my tweet from a couple of days earlier, he was telling me what I already knew – that to any reader other than me, I had failed to make my point, or much sense at all, for that matter.

'So what should I do – try speaking to Imani?'

'I'd *leave* it, man, I know it's tempting, but emotions running high, you're just going to make things worse. Give it time, I'm sure thing will cool off.'

This wasn't what I wanted to hear. The most narcissistic part of me can barely cope with being disliked. No part could handle being thought of as not caring about what was happening.

Knowing Leon was right, I thanked him, hung up, and proceeded to do the exact opposite of what he had advised.

'Hey, I can't stop thinking about that back and forth – I'd like the chance to chat about it properly if you're happy to – if at all possible, I'm keen to sort this out'.

I hit send. Given my recent track record firing off messages into the ether, I wasn't hopeful. To my surprise, however, I got a response from Imani almost instantly.

'Sure, I'm happy to do that – when's good for you?'

She wasn't giving much away, but also wasn't telling me to get lost, so not a total disaster.

* * *

The closer I got to Vauxhall, the more apparent it became that social distancing would be a farce. As the escalator carried me closer to the surface, the ticket hall was backed up from the crowd waiting to join the thousands already marching outside. Like a good boy scout, I had donned my FFP3, something that, early on in the pandemic, could still feel self-consciously over the top. Today, however, I didn't feel out of place among the kerchiefs, balaclavas and other makeshift face coverings.

When I got out into the not-so-open air, I had a voice note (a form of communication I am too calcified and prematurely geriatric in my ways to embrace) from Imani saying she was nearly there. Having made our peace, we had both agreed we felt compelled to be out, doing at least something in the real world.

The streets were an echo of that day protesting the war in 2003, but with a demographic shift reflecting the issue at hand, one that felt closer to home. Around me thronged activated young people. It's easy for commentators on the right to write protestors off as a mix of opportunistic troublemakers and misguided kids looking to fill an afternoon – but that ignores the energy that was obvious if you were there. A valve had been opened, releasing the frustration that can be so hard to articulate. Feelings of being leaned on by the weight of an establishment that doesn't value or respect you, that with its statues elevates figures who oppressed people like you.

As Imani approached, black aviator sunglasses, military boots and khaki lent a revolutionary aesthetic. Her braids were tied back and bound by a dark green knotted bandanna. By this point in the pandemic, the hug reflex had been beaten out of us all, and we went for the now terminally appropriated fist bump.

'Are you ready for this?'

'I think so . . .'

We merged into the stream – heading in the direction of the American embassy. How the British government managed to convince the US that Vauxhall, or more accurately the new-build explosion 'Nine Elms', was a suitably salubrious location for their diplomatic mission, and to move from Grosvenor Square I'm unsure – but it was a feat of persuasion.

I have friends who still treat a journey below the dividing line of the Thames as an adventure holiday, complete with the need for vaccination and travel insurance. Buttoned-up diplomats had traded the Georgian splendour of Mayfair for south of the river, with some of London's most notorious bacchanalian nightlife emporia as neighbours.

The walk was educational. As we moved, Imani managed to multitask with admirable skill. She simultaneously dodged bollards, lamp posts and other protestors, all while holding her phone aloft, looking down the barrel of the camera.

'So we're here at the protest – people are out, marching, being heard.'

She was live, broadcasting with the same level of comfort as if speaking to someone standing next to her – confident she'd get the tone right, not stumbling, paralysed by the thought the next sentence might be the misstep that would stir up an online posse.

The contrast between our respective levels of comfort and skill projecting our thoughts straight to the public was stark. The other distinction of course being that, given her exponentially greater number of followers, if she broadcast, people would actually be watching.

The roof of a bus shelter had been commandeered and acted as a podium. A group balanced on top, the elevated position apparently indicative of a higher level of commitment, and therefore status. Slogans echoed down from a young woman with long thin locks shouting into a loud hailer.

'No justice . . .'

In unison the crowd below responded.

'No peace!'

'Silence . . .'

'Is violence!'

Next to her a figure stood, eyes obscured by VR goggles, looking like an android programmed for progressive politics, his drone hovering overhead. It took off above the crowd, climbing slightly, before diving lower, filming to provide a counterpoint to the much-contested mainstream documentation of these events.

Transfixed, I almost failed to react when the ripple of someone taking the knee spread backwards like a Mexican wave, everyone dropping to the asphalt in solidarity. I joined them but, caught off guard by this sudden sincere display, moved with awkwardness almost matching the cringe-inducing images of Keir Starmer and other politicians, bent and appealing desperately to camera.

In another mirror to 2003, once the march reached the destination, it became a challenge to decide what to do. The momentum and purpose of direction can so easily dissipate into half-hearted chanting. This is still preferable to the alternative: kettled simmering frustration boiling over into confrontation and violence – in the process, the minority dominating the story and the front page.

Today, for the most part, it felt as if the former would prevail. We stood outside the embassy, a space-age cube encased in sail-like plastic, looking up at no one in particular. The day's refrains were recycled.

After another half an hour or so of this, Imani and I both sensed we had achieved all we could by being there. We joined the slipstream of like-minded people who now formed a loose convoy heading back along the river.

As we walked, the conversation served up a resolution, that if it appeared as dialogue in a straight-to-TV movie, might feel too neat and on the nose. Unpressured, we both acknowledged the Twitter exchange had gotten out of hand. I conceded that, even with the most charitable reading of my intent, the tweet had been completely incomprehensible. She reassured me the incendiary response was as much a result of the raw emotion of the moment as anything else.

Silence is violence – the phrase that became branded on the moment. This is undoubtedly true – it can do harm. After this episode, you might expect my social media output to have changed, chastened into posting about everything and anything I believe is important. But it's never going to be where I tell the world much about how I feel, or what I think – much as milestones like getting married and having a child have gone unannounced. The hypocrisy of still resorting to it for reasons of desperate self-promotion, however, while posting about nothing else, isn't lost on me.

I still experience Twitter (or X if you insist) and other social media as a churning slurry of anxiety, the (in this instance realised) fear something you say will be misunderstood, exploding in your face. And much of what's posted in solidarity can end up being meaningless. The sudden vocal and visible response from companies and celebrities scrabbling to show support has predictably dissolved back into nothingness – and worse with the widespread, cowardly rollback of diversity, equity and inclusion initiatives now the political wind has changed. The black squares that appeared were apparently sufficient stand-in for action and real change.

None of this is to devalue the benefit others derive from social media, the work that can be done there, the communities that have found and supported each other. Nor am I intending to project the air of superiority some do, when they smugly proclaim they don't use it – with the same tone as parents telling you their kids only play with wooden toys, never eat sugar and speak four languages. I just personally hate the experience, and refuse to make it a part of my daily life.

I'll admit, however, that I have yet to reconcile this with the fact it is where some of the most important conversations can happen, with the urgency and vitality missing elsewhere – and being absent from this is a problem. As I found, cutting yourself off from a network, its circuits, is to risk ignoring the most vital signs.

CHAPTER 16

Idols

HE HAD BEEN coughing for too long now. It wasn't COVID – multiple tests had come back negative, and at first it was the only symptom. Persuading a stoic man of his generation to go to the GP was always going to be a struggle, but he had finally submitted, and been sent straight to get a chest X-ray. In the often-languid timeframe of NHS investigation and treatment, this same-day urgency and concern isn't reassuring.

I was in the SpR office when my phone vibrated, Louise's name announced across the screen. It now feels as if when a call comes unexpectedly, something dramatic has happened – good or bad. Whatever the news, it's too urgent or serious for WhatsApp.

I stepped out into the July sun, immediately pacing along the fringes of the car park.

Uncharacteristically quiet, she was matter-of-fact.

'My dad's got a big pleural effusion on one side.'

In this short sentence there was so much. Anyone with a little knowledge would know this could never be good. A collection of fluid between the lining of the lung and the chest wall, there are many things that can cause an effusion. When the kidneys hang on to too much water – either because they're not working, or as part of the vicious cycle of heart failure – fluid accumulates on both sides.

Just on one side, however, it's almost always because something unpleasant is happening locally.

'It could still just be an infection.'

This was all the reassurance I could offer – an attempt for both of us to avoid jumping to what felt like the inevitable conclusion, but instead allowing ourselves to be pulled steadily through the process of investigation and gradual dismissal of more hopeful possibilities. As a GP, it would soon inevitably be Louise's job to explain everything to the rest of the family.

With this presentation, pneumonia would have perversely been the best possible outcome. But we both knew it wasn't that – it's pretty hard to have half a lung full of pus from an infection for this long and no fever.

He had never been a smoker, spending much of his youth playing serious football. He had, however, worked jobs that exposed him to the worst excesses of industrial and corporate negligence.

Despite it being known to be harmful since the start of the 20th century, asbestos was seemingly used for everything. Working as an engineer in the printing press of a notorious London paper, the whole place may as well have been made out of the stuff. The machine brakes were lined with it to counteract overheating, and there are stories of workers stuffing wads of raw white material into the parts. The innocent-seeming, cotton wool-like clouds filled the air with invisible, lethal microscopic fibres.

Armchair reactionaries love talking about health and safety

gone mad – but the alternative is to leave workers and the public at the mercy of injury for the sake of financial interests.

* * *

Meeting a father-in-law is always a roll of the dice. They are programmed for suspicion, and rightly so – given the sea of reprobates out there, a tide of dickheads that can never be held back, ranging from the relatively innocuous but unbearable soft boi your daughter meets in the first term at university, to the more dangerous. Fortunately, Edward (or Ted) was as relaxed and welcoming as you could ever hope for.

He had perfected moving with the flow of life, rather than struggling against it. Born in Tooting, he followed his father into the print, working there until a collision between the unions and bosses gutted the workforce.

Apparently, in the good old days, a machine was a machine – and a vehicle's engine not so different from a printing press. From then on, he made his living working on cars, fixing and selling them with a degree of small business success that might nowadays sound like a pipe dream.

Self-sacrificing in the most classically 'dad' way, the beneficiaries were his children. He was a man who, when his kids came to him with the home counties classic of 'we want a pony', didn't just double-, but quadruple-downed, and ended up owning and running a riding school.

This is how he ended up a rogue working-class voice among the at times absurd equine people, with their solariums and massages for pampered horses. By the time I met him, he was working on his own terms, when he wanted – a friend half teasing him that he was 'the most contented man in the world', surrounded by his family and busying himself with odd jobs around the yard.

In some ways I can relate to a sense of being out of place. The middle England surrounding London is a place I never feel wholly comfortable, feeling judged – as if the people are waiting to be impressed, having to prove my worth. Standing out, there's always that slight feeling of extra attention paid in shops, imagined or otherwise.

I lack one thing that would have endeared me to Ted – namely any real interest in football, and yet he nobly overlooked this. He would tolerate my inane questions and half-formed opinions if I ever hovered during *Match of the Day*.

* * *

He had been admitted to hospital for two nights, gradually settling into the retiree's summer camp experience that had sprung up with the other men in the bay. This atmosphere had been pierced early the first morning, when he'd been wheeled around to the procedure room amid a flurry of consent forms and concern.

If left untreated, the fluid has nowhere to go, and so builds up, gradually pressing on the many other important things you keep in your chest, like your heart. The answer is a pleural drain – inserting a vicious-looking spike, followed by silicone tubing through the chest wall.

Once the fluid had been drained – an experience he reliably informed us was 'fuckin' horrible', he was observed for another night. By the following day, he was champing for discharge. People often say they hate hospitals, which seems pretty redundant – few sane people like being there, at least not on the patient's side of the stethoscope.

Although what they had drained off would be sent for analysis, he would need a biopsy from the lining around the lung. He was assured this would happen in the next couple of weeks; they would contact him, and he was sent on his way. A word of advice: if you're expecting follow-up, never leave hospital without knowing how to get back in touch.

Sometimes admin can be the scariest, potentially most lethal component in healthcare – the cog that, if it fails, grinds everything to a halt. If you're not careful, you can be left in blissful ignorance, thinking the wheels are turning and progress is being made – only to find nobody has booked your next life-determining appointment.

By the next week, he hadn't heard anything, and by this point it was more than Louise could take. What followed was days on the phone trying to work out whose responsibility it was to fill in a simple request form to arrange the procedure. It became clear that nothing had been booked – an instance where, without pushy kids, a doctor no less, a patient would have languished untreated indefinitely.

* * *

Something you never appreciate about illness until you, or someone you care about, is ill, is how much waiting around there is. On the sofa, with little to do, he became an aficionado of daytime TV. We were both in the living room, letting the rolling BBC News wash over us. Now that a couple of months had passed since the peak of the George Floyd protests and statue-icide, a deeper reflection was going on. Retrospective pieces dissecting the sentiments and underlying reasons appeared.

There were high-profile acts of enthusiastic iconoclasm, and as the idols toppled, reactionary counter-movements had sprung up. The British Bulldog pints, carvery and Spitfire appreciation society gathered around monuments, promising to defend them –

their porcine skin flushed, glazed with sweat, crackling with 'patriotic' fury in the summer heat.

Medics are no strangers to being forced to reappraise and jettison celebrated figures. I have lost count of the number of diseases I have been forced to learn new names for, because they were discovered by someone who turned out to be a bad guy. In rheumatology, patients with 'Wegener's disease', a form of vasculitis (blood vessel inflammation), have had to rechristen their illness 'granulomatosis with polyangiitis' (rolls off the tongue), because, like a depressing number of notable physicians, Friedrich Wegener was a Nazi.

It is possible to reap the benefits of progress and achievement, without having to keep the shrine, if the idol proves unworthy. Of course, one alternative to toppling statues would be to augment them – with work that balances the story, depicting their worst moments and telling the other side of their story. In Whitehall, a new bronze of Churchill desperately clutching on to a sack of rice during the Bengal famine, for example.

The Winston Churchill fever that still grips much of Britain, I can in some small way understand. If that's your thing, he is at least the Nike, the Coke of historical 'great' white guys with terrible views and certain equally reprehensible actions to their names. He did know how to give a good speech, and by accounts walked the walk when it came to courage under fire. Some of the others being defended, however, make little sense – Colston and Cecil Rhodes are more blot than copy book. With colonialists, advocates often point to their supposed non-violent achievements, things like the railways, as if these were gifts to the indigenous populations. The trains were instruments, tools of efficiency that just allowed perpetrators to get to the oppression faster.

'Have you ever experienced much racism?'

I was taken back by Ted's question, for a couple of reasons. Firstly, we had almost never even skirted any deep topics. Secondly, I had forgotten that, for the most part, people just don't know – of course, every racialised person who has been on earth long enough, in a white majority country, has experienced racism, whether or not they care to admit it, or even realise it themselves.

Sometimes it is as simple as not having asked the question before. We continually overestimate the capacity of people to think about the problems of others – when, in reality, comfortable as any life may seem, most of us, most of the time, are struggling just to deal with what's in front of us that day.

It was a small thing, just to ask the question – but for him to at least remain curious, concerned even under the weight of his own predicament, mattered.

'Have I experienced racism? Where to start? Chronologically, or in order of severity?'

(I of course didn't say this.)

* * *

I have seen idols toppled in real time during my medical career. Consultants who were untouchable sidelined, and in some cases exiled altogether. Sometimes it was because of their behaviour, but often they were simply themselves victims of university politics. The bad actor's comeuppance merely collateral damage in the fallout from a colleague's ambition.

At medical school, with third year comes the opportunity to really get into the shit. Being unleashed on the wards, the chance to gain some clinical skills, but also placing you fully at the mercy of the egomaniacs and despots that still haunt many of the hospitals.

One name, prior to his fall, was enough to conjure a chill.

A nephrologist by trade, among the medical consultants, Dr Garside was the most enthusiastic when it came to enforcing sleep deprivation. He would roll-call for his dawn ward round that followed our mandated night shift, making sure to hunt down any missing names. While not unfamiliar with being up at this time after being awake all night, this was the first any of us had been forced to do it sober. One encounter, as a student in 2010, will never leave me.

'So, what, you thought a fucking cardiac arrest was more important than my ward round?'

This is a challenging question to answer, because, in many ways, the short answer would be yes – certainly if you asked the patient they'd say so. We had been advised by the medical SpR to stay and watch the A&E team in their attempts to break the rib cage of (resuscitate) a middle-aged man found collapsed, likely from a massive coronary.

'Think you've got more to learn from watching some poor bastard shuffle off this mortal coil than from me?'

He had only the slightest hint of Scottish to his voice, the kind of confusing accent produced by their boarding schools. At this moment, it was charged with fury, but not yet full and unrestrained. More silence from us – although perhaps he had a point on this front; the level of aggression in his teaching style meant that you *did* tend to remember *anything* he taught you, it just might be as you awoke in a cold sweat from a night terror.

Dr Garside's black, swept-back hair created a sense of motion, as if he was accelerating towards you, and the twitching bristle of his magician's goatee insinuated that whatever he did when he arrived might be unsavoury. Medical students and doctors alike were right to be wary of him, as he was a renowned 'challenging character'. Unfortunately, he was also clever – to the wide-eyed and naive among us seemingly bordering on genius, and usually correct when it comes to medicine, so he got away with it.

This is a man who, during a lecture, displayed an image demonstrating the effects of leprosy and pronounced of the subject's dark skin: 'Looks like I found him swinging through the jungles of Africa.'

Nevertheless, his talks were religiously attended, because if there is one thing medical students prize above social justice, it's exam success. Alongside work on the wards, his lab maintained an impressive research output, and most importantly to us, he set many of the exam questions we'd face at the end of the year. Even now, I'm embarrassed to say my feelings remain more mixed than they should be. I have undoubtedly learned a huge amount from him, but at what cost?

The post-take ward round is an archaic circus of a tradition that occurs every morning, where the night medical team attempt to round up the intake of patients – and justify their nocturnal actions to the boss. The first and often most difficult task is finding them, as although in theory they should move seamlessly from A&E to the acute medical unit, often, they do not. Because the hospital is full, instead they often end up as 'outliers' in some strange part of the hospital, forgotten and unloved.

When the post-take consultant is Dr Garside, preparation is everything. The medical registrar had better know the route this safari round is taking – or else risk the lament: 'I knew you could barely read a medical textbook, but I would have hoped you could at least read a map of the fucking hospital.'

This will then set the tone for the session on the rack to follow at the patient's bedside. The helpless house officer might find themselves on the receiving end of the following:

'Why did you give this patient a diuretic?'

'Because I think her shortness of breath is because of heart failure.'

'But you just told me a minute ago she had pneumonia on the chest X-ray.'

'Yes.'

'Well, which is it?'

'Um . . . both?'

'How many diagnoses do you want? One?' As he said this, he held up the middle finger of one hand (the impolite way). 'Or two?' At this point the first middle finger was joined by that of the other hand.

This morning, at least he had swept in jovially (by his standards), rather than all-out malicious. Us not all being present and waiting for the start of the sacred ritual had been a wobble, but not terminal – in that he hadn't sent us away in fury.

'Right, let's get on with this magical misery tour – where are you taking me first?'

'Shall we start in ED?'

'I don't know, shall we? You don't sound sure.'

Ruth, the medical SpR, hesitantly confirmed: 'Yes, there are a couple still down there.'

At that, the site of his first sacrifice confirmed, he strode ahead, energised at the prospect of drawing blood.

The first splash of cold water was not a comment about a doctor or student, but a patient. Behind the curtain – the flimsy, readily moveable shield protecting the patient's dignity from the gawping masses outside – we huddled nervously around a bewildered-looking man in his forties.

'So you've been feeling a bit breathless? When was the last time you saw your cardiologist?'

'It's been a while – probably coming up to a year.'

'Well *he* probably should be keeping a closer eye on you. We'll let him know you're in.'

Dr Garside was of course not above passing judgement on the perceived failings of colleagues – in the presence of patients and students alike. He proceeded to snap in his stethoscope earpieces, and delicately placed the diaphragm on the chest, eyes closed like a virtuoso musician channelling the heart sounds.

'S1 + S2 + S3.'

He rattled off the presence of the two normal beats, and the third sound indicating this one was less than happy, possibly medically broken.

Out of earshot, he grilled Laura, one of the students in our group: 'Now, what drug has caused that man's gynaecomastia?'

'His gynaecomastia . . .'

'His tits! He had the biggest pair in the room!'

She stared at him blankly.

Losing his patience: 'Spironolactone, it's called spironolactone – Christ help the patients of tomorrow.'

The point at which the ward round took a fatal nosedive had nothing to do with medicine, or hospital geography. As we walked past a poster of Maria Alvarez (who was Filipina – don't worry, that's relevant), the hospital's head nurse, he slowed and a half-smile crept out from underneath the canopy covering his top lip.

He turned and asked one of the other medical students, Soo-Jin (who was Korean): 'Relative of yours?'

I'm not sure he expected an answer, and he was rewarded with exactly that, silence – the thundering silence of everyone else in the group's heads simultaneously exploding, while we all said nothing.

Having detonated that, he quickened his pace and we followed open-mouthed in his wake towards his next victim.

Although extreme, this encounter isn't unique. Experience of racism among doctors is widespread – to the point it is almost universal among ethnic minority staff. When the BMA asked, 91 per cent of black respondents reported they had experienced racism at work. Accepting the limitations of a survey, most would agree that's a lot.

Trainees described being treated differently from their white colleagues by supervising consultants and other staff. They are more likely to face close scrutiny and be criticised. There are enough dinosaurs still roaming the hospitals, whose retro views influence which students they prey on, for bullying to create a hostile learning environment. This is likely to impact attainment. You're less likely to sit through a lecture, where precious mark-winning pearls are dispensed, if the lecturer seasons it with their hot takes on racial theory.

The effect of this is, of course, compounded if you are either a non-UK medical graduate with an 'accent' (as if everyone doesn't have one) or, surprising no one, a woman.

Dr Garside stayed around far longer than he should have – but even he wasn't bulletproof. Eventually, he was apparently quietly asked to perhaps take a sabbatical, but decided there were far more lucrative opportunities than academia and left the university entirely. Although gone, it does feel as if being put out to pasture in a field of cash is hardly comeuppance.

* * *

The results of Ted's biopsy were no surprise, but still, all at once crushing. Mesothelioma is a cancer the first Google hit described as having a 'dismal' prognosis. Although perhaps accurate, this is hardly a morale boost when the patient or their family first read it.

As a doctor, when a family member is sick, you can struggle to be rational and scientific about things. Even when a symptom is almost certainly nothing, you're vigilant for the worst. However, when presented with catastrophe, despite the impersonal brutish cudgel of statistics, if there is any hope, then many among us will still seek it out and cling to it like a raft in a cyclone.

He was relatively young, and otherwise fit and healthy – he might have been among the 5 per cent on the sunny side of the slope of the survival curve. Offered the choice of where to be treated, Louise and my advice (insistence) was the specialist hospital with the headline-bothering academics. While no doubt the care at the local place is great, the instinct is that when you have something rare and horrible, it's a good idea to get as close to the eggheads as possible.

COVID added unwelcome layers of complexity to a cancer diagnosis. It's useful to have another person with you at hospital appointments when it's something serious – someone who may at least be marginally less stunned by the whole situation, able to focus enough to ask for further explanations, or prompt you to report new symptoms.

None of this was possible for much of the summer and autumn of 2020. My mother-in-law would drop Ted off, like a kid at the school gates. He had to go in and face whatever was coming that day alone – the information and emotional torrent of new results and treatment options. And, of course, cancer treatment is complicated and confusing – understanding what a Positron Emission Tomography CT does, what new 'areas of activity' on the scan mean, and the reasons why surgery isn't possible.

'What did the doctor say?' would often be met with frustrating vagueness.

Medical students get whole lectures dedicated to understanding why we may give a patient immunotherapy, how it works. But he was expected to sign on to it without support in understanding why it was his best chance at living longer.

He dealt with it all admirably, but the changes were painfully quick. The descent in illness moves in a spiral, the radius of the world shrinking as the energy to venture out becomes too much. As quickly as he changed, the days slowed.

This was amplified by the ever-shifting restrictions – dictating where he could go, who could visit. There was also the prevalence, and the reality, that he was the very definition of high risk. With every decision by his daughter, his grandchildren, to come and spend what may be some of their last time together, there was the background hum of fear.

And then, just as quickly, the dreadful suspended waiting was suddenly replaced. We were irresistibly pulled down through loss and into grief. It feels absurd, childish even, to talk about fair – Louise and I have both seen enough to know that doesn't come into it. But it isn't fair he was made ill because employers and those policing them didn't care enough, isn't fair he didn't make it to the wedding we had hastily arranged in the hope he'd be there, and that our daughter won't ever get to meet him.

It can be tempting to sum a person up, grasp at conclusions and lessons after something senseless. But if I could, I'd take from him a Zen-like ability to accept change and adapt to life – and to be contented, rather than chasing some elevated status or imagined legacy, other than the one left to your family.

CHAPTER 17

Misinformation

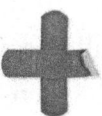

AT TIMES, HONESTY can dent the confidence of patients and their families – especially when you admit you're not sure what's going on.

'We don't know what's wrong – but I promise, we're doing *everything* we can to find out.'

This is about as reassuring as seeing your pilot cramming *The Idiot's Guide to Aviation* as you board the plane.

On this occasion, Kyle, a 21-year-old man, had come in with an illness we couldn't explain, and his condition was becoming ever more precarious. It had started with itchy purple rashes all over his body, soon followed by fevers. Now his heart was sprinting, while his blood pressure was slumped lazily in the region of 90 systolic and he was needing an increasingly worrying amount of oxygen.

His admission swab had been negative for COVID – although around this time, there was a widespread feeling that everything was being blamed on the virus. Prices in the shop gone up?

COVID. Project delayed? COVID. Louise asking why I haven't taken the bins out? COVID.

Doctors weren't immune from this – it felt like there weren't any other illnesses coming into the hospital. When a strange new disease has the entire world in its grip, it's tempting to blame it for anything weird that shows up. This wasn't always wide of the mark – when people started getting painful, purple chilblain rashes on their feet, this imaginatively became known as 'COVID toes', a suspicion that eventually proved correct.

We couldn't be sure, and when a young person is this sick and you don't have an answer, not keeping an open mind can be lethal. It could be an infection you've just not found yet, or that euphemistic 'something sinister' – lymphoma or some other cancer.

He was in the 'clean' section of the HDU, which meant we were spared the beekeeper suits and the visiting rules were more relaxed. His body had been running a marathon while lying still – he was exhausted and so he slept. His father was sitting by his bedside, keeping vigil.

He had already been woken up several times in the past hour or so, and I wasn't going to add much by prodding him into consciousness again. I settled for what can be a surprisingly useful assessment – just taking a look. His heart and breathing, although not normal, hadn't gotten any worse; the machines hadn't added any new alarms to their chorus.

His dad didn't seem much older than me – although given the age of his child, we had clearly spent our time *very* differently during our teenage years. We were both black men in our 30s, careering towards middle age, and had found some common ground, the foundations for small talk over the past couple of days.

I asked the standard: 'How are you doing? Have you got any questions?'

'What do you think about the idea the vaccines could be bad for you?'

I didn't immediately answer, waiting to see where this was going – so he continued.

'And people are saying they made the virus so they could inject people?'

When soliciting questions, a trip into tin-foil-hat land wasn't quite what I had in mind.

If ever there were a time to be diplomatic . . . but also, if the answer *was* 'yes', was he *really* expecting the frontman of a global conspiracy to be honest? A sudden lapse in secrecy with my guard down blowing the whole thing wide open?

'Well . . . all medicines aren't completely risk-free . . . but with the vaccine, for almost everyone, the benefit outweighs the risks.'

He nodded, more in understanding than agreement, and seemed to be weighing the words. I don't think his mind had been made up one way or the other – whatever I said was hardly likely to cast the deciding vote.

I almost didn't need to add 'and definitely no mind control' (not a side effect medical school had prepared me to have to reassure patients about).

As if musing to himself as much as speaking to me, he added: 'But they *do* just want to control people.'

This sentiment, although misidentified with vaccines and a potential malicious origin of COVID, is understandable. Suddenly being locked inside, and warned not to associate with others because of an invisible threat, one that experts were struggling to explain the origins of, feels like control. Police patrolled parks as if ready to check your Fitbit to ensure you were really exercising, food in pubs and restaurants was measured to determine if it met the 'substantial meal' test to allow for an alcoholic drink.

It didn't help that, early in the pandemic, councils used the opportunity of deserted streets to roll out new measures, like low-traffic neighbourhoods. To be clear, I'm on board with the utopian aims of making walking and cycling more pleasant and reducing pollution. Enough was done badly, however, to piss people off. I have the suspicion that some local town planning departments are not awash with talent, overflowing with good ideas. I have seen enough murderously over-optimistic bike lanes painted onto road space still used by cars.

There was a feeling that the changes simultaneously inconvenienced those forced to still go out to work, such as delivery drivers, while also arbitrarily pushing traffic away from more affluent residential areas – towards places where more disadvantaged groups live. Mistrust at the motivations, coupled with the timing, meant anger evolved. Over the years that followed, something that sounds as pleasant as the '15-minute' city – where residents can reach the majority of destinations quickly, without a car, became a beacon for conspiratorial thinking.

Personally, I'd love it – I live in London, where a commute often means practically tasting the sweat of fellow travellers, packed in conditions that would be illegal for livestock. And yet these neighbourhoods have been reimagined as the 'open-air prisons' of 'the Great Reset', with residents banned from leaving their designated sector – the post-COVID world envisioned by supposed shadowy, gilet-clad elites, their spectral hands manipulating events from their Davos lair.

It is difficult to discuss conspiracy theories, without addressing the ethnic and racial scapegoating that often comes with them. Dangerous, delusional beliefs about Jews are as old as anti-semitism itself – and any time the word 'globalist' or 'elite' is used, there is the worry that this is code for what is really meant.

At the same time, white nationalists fear the white populations of European countries and North America being replaced by migrants from African and Muslim majority countries elsewhere. These two hatreds fuse in the minds of neo-Nazi extremists like Callum Parslow, who in April 2024 stabbed an asylum seeker from Eritrea, believing that boat crossings were part of this 'Great Replacement' – orchestrated by those very 'elites'.

Black and other non-white UK residents were more likely to feel the force of COVID enforcement. Across the country, black people were three times more likely to face fines, and in Cumbria, those from an ethnic minority background were eight times as likely compared to White British counterparts. It is understandable how this could make fertile soil – to sow the idea that the pandemic was just an excuse to further oppress an overpoliced people.

Marginalised groups can be more at risk of influence from dangerous conspiracy theories. Dangerous, because they can further dent members' ability to derive maximum benefit and thrive in society. This has nothing to do with intelligence, and the reasons are complex, but a significant part is due to legitimate suspicion of traditional authorities and institutions, including the medical establishment.

Throughout the 20th century, there have been several instances of medical practitioners conducting unethical research and forcing 'treatment' on non-white groups. The most famous is the Tuskegee Syphilis Study in the US, running from 1932 to 1972. In Alabama, that bastion of racial equity, African American sharecroppers were observed, to document the natural course of syphilis infection.

Syphilis is a sexually transmitted infection caused by the pig-tail shaped bacterium Treponema pallidum. The prevailing 'Columbian' theory is that this infection has been with humans in the Americas (not that the inhabitants were calling them that) for thousands of years. Spanish conquistadors, doing what colonisers do best, screwing the indigenous inhabitants (literally, as well as figuratively), picked it up along with gold on their travels, bringing it back to Europe as a weeping genital penance for their actions.

The disease went on to ravage Europe from the 15th century onwards, crippling armies and burning through society. If you set aside the human misery and suffering (which you probably shouldn't), it is a fascinating disease.

Occurring in several stages, from the early ulcers of the initial infection, through a dormant period, it can then pop up, like an unkillable slasher villain years later, as tertiary syphilis – damaging the heart or nervous system. Along with lupus and TB, it is an entry on my top-tip list for medical students of diseases that can cause pretty much anything. The manifestations have been luridly documented countless times in literature and art, the afflicted portrayed in paintings and poetry.

A wealth of previous observational evidence existed that syphilis was, medically speaking, bad news. Despite this, Tuskegee study coordinators apparently felt it would be beneficial to continue to study the effects of the disease left untreated. This went on long after an effective cure, penicillin, became widely available – and many participants went on to die of the disease, sacrificed to medical curiosity.

In Tuskegee, contrary to popular belief, unwitting patients weren't deliberately infected with syphilis. US doctors reserved those experiments for subjects in a country where they would face even less scrutiny – Guatemala. The two 'studies' did share an important cast member, however. John Charles Cutler was born in Cleveland, Ohio, in 1915 and graduated medical school in

1941, coming of age professionally the year America entered the Second World War.

Commissioned into the US Public Health Service, he would have been all too aware of the potential for VD to derail D-Day. Stinging, weeping genitals can be a distraction when storming a Normandy beach. During the war he studied inmates at the penitentiary in Terre Haute, Indiana – participants 'consented' to being deliberately infected with a smorgasbord of clap (varied preparations of gonorrhoea) in exchange for cash and favourable recommendations to the parole board. It is of course debatable whether a prisoner under these circumstances can truly consent.

Between 1946 and 1948, he graduated in his ambitions, increasing the magnitude of his ethical violations. Taking his ideas on tour, in Guatemala he infected un-consenting victims including orphaned children, psychiatric inpatients and prisoners with syphilis and gonorrhoea. Some of the descriptions of the methods are gruesome, and sound like something out of a *Saw* film. They included direct spinal injections of bacteria, and inoculation of pus into the eyes – practices which, had he found himself on the losing side in a war, might have meant he had a few more questions to answer.

Far from being made a pariah for these crimes (and they were morally, if not legally, considered crimes by the time of the study's end; the Nuremberg Code was written in 1947), he enjoyed a celebrated career, being appointed assistant Surgeon General of the US Public Health Service in 1958.

Apparently, the world of monstrous venereal disease research is small – and he would go on to join the Tuskegee study in the 1960s. Unrepentant later in life, he maintained that the study and its methods were essential, carried out with the interests of public health in the black community at heart. He can be seen affirming this in the 1993 PBS Nova documentary *Deadly Deception* – at the time of writing still available in all its crackly audio, pastel-coloured glory on YouTube.

Bad news travels, and often the global African diaspora looks to the US for cultural cues. These experiments have undoubtedly damaged trust in the medical establishment internationally. This supplements an already healthy mistrust of authority (of which, like it or not, we as medical practitioners are representatives) among the descendants of colonised people.

In the UK, although nothing quite on this scale has been perpetrated, we are not unblemished when it comes to unethical experimentation. In 1969, researchers in Coventry fed women chapatis containing radioactive iron, apparently without their knowledge (exacerbated by a lack of translation, as many subjects didn't speak English), in order to investigate the causes of anaemia. Aside from the obvious disregard for basic ethics, the tainting and subversion of food, and therefore culture, in the process of abusing participants feels especially perverse.

Organisations in the modern era whose values many pro-gressives agree with, can also suffer through association with perceived bad actors. In the US, Planned Parenthood has been vital in securing and maintaining access to family planning, including abortion. It's hardly surprising, however, that the founder Margaret Sanger's links to the Eugenics movement have raised a few questions. The organisation has had to defend itself against the accusation it was established to control the birth rates of minority groups. It has been alleged that clinics are preferentially placed in black neighbourhoods to help keep numbers low.

Even if this theory were true, when it comes to methods of oppression, this would turn out to be a pretty dumb approach. All of the evidence suggests that access to safe and effective

family planning is one of the best ways of raising women out of
poverty – and I'm not sure enabling black female social mobility
is high on the agenda for the racial purists.

Historical gynaecologists don't get off scot-free, however. It
is true that throughout the 20th century, in other instances, US
doctors sterilised a great many black women against their will, for
what were clearly spurious reasons – labelling them as mentally
inadequate, delinquent or otherwise unfit. A great deal has been
written on this – and in the first instance I would point you in the
direction of Dr Annabel Sowemimo's *Divided*.

* * *

Young people who look like they're careening in the wrong
direction put everyone on edge, particularly when you throw in
a medical mystery. You can find yourself eventually just gazing
blindly at the numbers – willing the blood pressure to come up,
the heart rate to come down.

Kyle and his fever had been steaming away for days now –
and everyone was all too aware that this could only go on for
so long. Bodies tire and hearts fail. We had called in everyone –
the infection doctors had been round, supplying plenty of
chin-stroking and a list of infection tests to send off. Likewise, we
had enlisted my bosses in rheumatology and added our specialty's
set menu of autoantibodies to the mix.

It was time to bite the bullet and give something. We were
fairly confident by this point that it was all being driven by
the immune system throwing a tantrum – an overreaction to the
recent COVID.

'We think we need to give some steroids.'

'Steroids? Like body builders take . . .'

This is a response so common we could do with an 'FAQ'

sheet – people imagining we're swelling their muscles to fight off the illness.

'Not exactly – more like the ones we give for asthma. They dampen down the immune system, and stops it attacking the body.'

Of course, if we were wrong, and he did have an infection, then we risked making things a lot worse – the medical equivalent of shelling your own troops mid-battle.

The other issue in situations like this, is that steroids can interfere with the diagnosis of blood disorders – temporarily shrinking that plump lymph node harbouring all the answers. But, as a rule of thumb, it's better to be alive with a little uncertainty than dead with a firm diagnosis.

The family agreed with the decision, the bag was hung and we waited. Fortunately for all of us, over the next days, his fevers improved, his heart rate slowed, and none of us would have to be answering questions in front of a judge. There was no infection; his immune system had been fighting phantom invaders.

* * *

'Do you believe all this then, do you?'

Headphones glued in, lost in the half-waking state of the perma-podcast listener, I didn't immediately understand the question.

She gestured at the mask covering my face.

'This rubbish, do you believe it?'

Not twice in one week, surely? Behind the counter, the weary middle-aged Turkish guy who had saved us all in the great toilet roll shortage of the early pandemic, when the big supermarket shelves were bare, rolled his eyes. Why couldn't she just let me get on with my post on-call shift, off-licence panic shop? This is a place you can get anything – including, on this occasion, herb-flecked flatbreads of improbable proportions.

'It depends, what you mean? Do I believe in COVID?'

She was a woman perhaps in her early 50s, with a mess of hair like frayed hessian compressed under a lilac woollen hat. The pompoms that dangled from the drooping ear flaps bobbed and swung as she spoke animatedly. She continued on, her monologue primed, whatever my reaction had been.

'I can show you a video of a Nobel Prize winner who knows what's really going on . . . and the man who invented PCR says it should never have been used for testing like this – all false positives.'

Where to start. The truest thing ever said about conspiracy theorists is that it's almost impossible to argue with them. Having settled into their chosen niche, they will have pressed their nose into every inch. They will undoubtedly 'know' more than you – even if this knowledge is complete horse shit. Satisfactorily rebuffing an individual point could take hours of research – you'll quickly sink in the slurry of nonsense.

She waved her phone under my nose, as a buffering video loaded – it was 90 minutes long. It was titled something like 'world leading Nobel scientist reveals the inside truth!'. Frustrated, she continued the rant.

'What do you believe then?!'

'I believe there is virus, that it causes COVID-19 . . . and in evidence that comes from properly conducted research and clinical trials.'

Her zeal turned to anger.

'Oh right, you're one of them, are you?! Already part of it . . . One day there's going to be a reckoning.'

This threat – of mass Nuremberg-style trials of medical professionals and politicians complicit in perpetrating the COVID 'conspiracy' – lurks beneath the surface of any conversation with believers. The logic apparently being, that in years to come, evidence that vaccines have caused an increase in deaths will come out – ideally coupled with proof there never was a virus anyway.

What isn't immediately clear, is how the invisible cabal responsible is sufficiently powerful to orchestrate a global pandemic – but would lack the IT skills to change the numbers on the Office for National Statistics website, to hide this spike in mortality.

Apparently threats of mass murder were where the owner drew the line – the point where it becomes bad for business. She had already been in the shop when I arrived, presumably firing off her spiel at anyone straying close – and didn't look like she was planning on leaving of her own accord any time soon.

'Okay, that's enough.'

'Yes, we have all had enough!'

'No, you need to leave.'

'Why?! You can't make me!'

He had the fixed, unmoving expression of a man who spends 14 hours a day standing behind the counter of a 24-hour offie in Catford, and has seen it all – the strip-light glow a beacon in the night for all manner of madness the streets have to offer.

'Don't make me call the police.'

'That's right – keep us all in line!'

Despite this vocal objection, she didn't seem up for a fight and shuffled angrily to the exit. The owner permitted himself the closest I have ever seen to a smile from him. I thanked him, paid for the bread and left.

For the most part, the people I see and speak to at work continue to trust doctors and the healthcare system. But it is impossible to go back; the trust in mainstream medicine is less absolute, which, although perhaps not all bad, does change the dynamic.

Ever more patients arrive in the clinic armed with advice and test results from alternative sources and healthcare providers. When discussing a new treatment, there will be more questions about the safety, and more questions about motives.

CHAPTER 18

No Woman No Cry

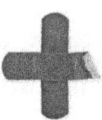

AT THE RISK of sounding like a tedious nerd, among the greatest advances to occur during my time working in hospitals, is electronic patient notes. There is now some hope that an accurate record of what has happened to you in hospital actually exists. No more illegible doctors' handwriting hieroglyphics to decipher, no pages falling out of the brick of notes – unintentionally or otherwise.

Once staff get used to it, the online drug chart is also no doubt safer – the risk of a lethal missed decimal point is drastically reduced, and the system carries helpful drug dosing prompts to prevent us from accidentally euthanising our patients with ten times the correct dose. Interaction warnings flash up if the combination of medications we're prescribing risk concocting a chemical car bomb inside the patient.

Not to say there aren't teething problems – whenever they are introduced, initially things slow down, especially in the clinics, like gumming up the gears in a machine. Often older, less digitally addicted staff, who didn't spend their adolescence hanging out on MSN Messenger, struggle more with the transition. In the most severe cases, I know of consultants for whom the introduction was the final nail, the change that knocked them into retirement.

I recall during the rollout of a new all-in-one system, an inpatient ward round was brought to a standstill by the boss's hissy fit, triggered by the challenges of the new patient record. His red face like an angry testicle, he paced back and forth, hands waving theatrically, because the blood test graphs looked different, his delicate equilibrium upset.

'Right, that's it, I'm not continuing until you go and find the patient's paper notes we were using yesterday.'

The wide-eyed 'floorwalker' – the IT support staff assigned to roam the wards fighting fires – was batted down the second he stepped up to offer help. The sister in charge of the ward had smiled uncomfortably.

'You *know* we can't do that.'

'Well then, we'll all just stand here,' he sandbagged like an angry toddler.

Eventually, only after he realised the stalemate would risk delaying his clinic – and presumably the private work he was planning after – he relented.

Errors are still of course possible – there have been headlines about deaths where electronic systems have contributed. But we know about these, at least in part, because they can be interrogated – paper notes were murky depths that guarded their secrets more closely.

A potentially unhealthy habit that access to patient notes everywhere in the hospital can foster is keeping tabs, like a parent hovering over the baby monitor. At any one time, I'll have a cohort I'm checking in on. This may be for educational purposes, learning what has happened to someone I have treated; just as often, however, it's my anxiety trying to ensure I haven't killed anyone – eyes flicking continually to the 'alive' or 'deceased' column next to their name.

* * *

The call had come from the obstetric team, which is a jolt that always bypasses all other body systems and heads straight to the gut.

'She's thirty-two weeks pregnant, and has COVID . . .'

It had been well established by this point that the two things didn't mix. Pregnancy is arguably an 'immune-compromised' state, throughout which instructions are sent to the immune system to take a chill pill, to prevent it from attacking the little bundle of joy/unwelcome guest (delete as appropriate).

While good for the passenger, this has the unwanted side effect of leaving the mother at increased risk of infection. This is the logic behind our practice of depriving pregnant women the delights of soft cheeses and sushi throughout (were the shoe on the other foot, these would no doubt be among my greatest struggles while expecting). This sedated immune system also didn't seem alert to COVID until it was too late – and young people who would otherwise have been in a low-risk group were getting really sick.

'She's on 60 per cent oxygen, and sats are only just hovering around 93 per cent.'

The obstetric registrar was saying all of this calmly, in a tone that was mismatched with the dread that had let itself in and was making itself comfortable in my chest. While we naturally want the best for all patients, the prospect of being responsible for a bad outcome in a mother and baby adds another few atmospheres of pressure.

That the average medic is poorly equipped to understand and manage the altered physiology of pregnancy is increasingly recognised. Alongside the sporadic updates and training days we get on the subject, an increasing number of doctors, both from the medical specialties and obstetrics side, are choosing to sub-specialise in maternal medicine.

They take on responsibility for helping to adapt the management of pre-existing conditions, because many treatments are untested or unsafe in pregnant women, and alternatives have to be found. They also deal with the unexpected curveballs pregnancy can throw – like type-2 diabetes in previously healthy women, and heart disease.

'I'll come, but I'm telling you now, she's going to need ITU, and I don't think there's much I can add before she gets moved there.'

This wasn't me shirking responsibility – as well as the immune considerations, in intelligent design terms, the mechanics of pregnancy haven't been very well thought through. Under normal (at least as far as we non-baby-catching medics are concerned) circumstances, respiration works through a combination of chest wall muscles moving your ribcage out, and the diaphragm immediately below your lungs pulling them down.

Even before they're born, kids get in the way – demanding extra oxygen, while simultaneously changing the physics of the whole process. Dealing with this in a woman with severe COVID wasn't something I was equipped for. But I went – mainly to confirm my suspicion that I'd be about as much use as a face mask with a kissing hole – and ensure that they were going to call someone who could actually help.

The obstetric unit is a troublingly long walk from the rest of the wards, to an area of the hospital that's otherwise deserted at night – meaning it's both a long way there in an emergency, and far away from the rest of the hospital where the rest of my work was waiting. The first is perhaps less of an issue, as the labour ward anaesthetists should be able to get to, and run, any maternal arrest in the time it takes me to puff along the forbidding corridor. Heading there to give a medical opinion, on the other hand, means abandoning the rest of the hospital.

Crashing around a maternity unit in the middle of the night doesn't endear you to anyone; they are notoriously impossible places to get any rest. Before the birth, in the early stages (particularly if you have an induction), you might be sharing a room. Afterwards, often in bays of four, with partners coming in and out and the new arrivals waking one another up whenever they get hungry, the problem is magnified further.

'Mrs Senaratne, I'm Matt, one of the medical doctors. I'm here to see how you're getting on.'

This felt more than a little redundant. We both knew she was in trouble – not even the most upbeat kids' TV presenter could put a positive spin on it.

She was receiving almost as much oxygen as it was possible to give her without intubation – and with that she was panting like she was actually giving birth there and then.

'I feel . . . tired . . .'

Again, not surprising – at 33 weeks, I'm reliably informed that's the baseline.

'Okay, we need to give you some more oxygen, but I think you might need to go and spend some time with my colleagues on intensive care.'

I tried to pitch it as un-alarmingly as possible, but perhaps ended up making it sound like she would be going on a mini break.

'Intensive care . . . Is my . . . baby . . . going to be . . . okay?'

Realistically, the answer to this was probably yes – she was far enough along that even in the case where delivery became necessary, the baby would be fine. But everything was weird with COVID, and there was no telling whether some unforeseen complication would pop up now, or weeks down the line.

Outside of wartime, COVID no doubt must have been the worst period in recent history to be pregnant. During this already anxiety-inducing and stress-filled time, a global pandemic now meant that stepping out of your home presented an impossible-to-quantify risk to your baby. Attending appointments, and even giving birth with restrictions in place, meant some women were having to face all pregnancy could throw at them alone.

I dusted off what I felt was my most reassuring tone.

'It'll be fine – the obstetric doctors and ICU team will take great care of you.'

I called the obstetric SpR – she was now somewhere else entirely, which is fair enough. When you might be called to go and yank out a baby at a moment's notice, it's unreasonable for anyone to expect you to hang around in one place.

'I mean, you can give her some nasal high flow here while you wait, but like I said, she needs to go to ICU.'

And that was the end of my direct involvement – turning up, stating the obvious, and then leaving.

* * *

The medical on-call rota just as quickly sling-shots you back to the 'normal' routine of your medical day job. I was back in my clinic room, with the discolouring paint on the walls, chipped wooden school desk and antique steam-powered PC. A lot of our appointments were still telephone consultations, which when it came to assessing joints were pretty pointless – unless your patient assured you that they felt so good they were considering taking up breakdancing.

But this format, and the relatively shorter length of time appointments took, did allow for more time gazing out of the window into the car park. With the wonders of the electronic notes, I could also stay up to date with the stories from my on-calls – checking repeatedly, waiting for them to refresh like social media.

I could see when they were forced to deliver the baby by C-section. I could see how, still intubated, they took her to ITU, the days she spent completely unconscious, followed by the slow waking and switch to a tracheostomy.

Her first few weeks of motherhood were about as abnormal as it was possible for them to be. After being released from hospital, the baby was staying with her husband's family. With some difficulty, but helped by the nurses, she was expressing milk – and when she was strong enough, the baby was brought in for longer and longer visits.

Her story, and how it would end, became entwined with the pandemic, the state of the world as a whole. I felt as if a bad outcome would mean the end of hope. Reading the daily entries, I sensed it must have been like living in a horror film for her and her family – in another language, with bad subtitles. They all spoke varying levels of English – magnifying the uncertainty and the fear.

Along with her, I could breathe easier when they started weaning the tracheostomy. Even more so when she was stepped down to the ward, and was reunited with her baby. She was eventually discharged as well as could be expected, but with what you can only imagine being the mother of all cases of long COVID.

* * *

Pregnancy and the post-partum period are unlikely to be a picnic for anyone – regardless of how special your experience, or how privileged they may be. After nine months of being drained like a power pack, then giving birth, or having major abdominal surgery, you're expected to offer round-the-clock room service to the most demanding of customers.

For non-white mothers, the experience is often worse, and the most objective and miserable measure of this is maternal mortality. The exact figures vary according to the sources and year studied, but the relative risk of death for black women during childbirth was in the recent past five times higher than for their white counterparts. The figures are similarly elevated for some other ethnic groups, for example Pakistani and Bangladeshi women – mirroring the disparities seen with COVID-19 infections. Importantly disparities persist even after controlling for income.

Morbidity and mortality have been attributed to a collage of factors, but the glue that binds them (predictably at this point) is racial bias. There are well-worn ideas about black people being able to tolerate more pain, so being offered less analgesia and fewer epidurals – interventions which have themselves been associated with improving maternal outcomes.

Other worrying symptoms may be dismissed – including those associated with the most common cause of death: blood clots. The talismanic example of this comes from the US. Serena Williams, despite being a multimillionaire, presumably able to afford the Rolls-Royce of deliveries, almost died when doctors ignored her concerns that she was developing a pulmonary embolism after giving birth. Candice Brathwaite gives a first person account of her concerns regarding a C-section wound infection being similarly dismissed – and the resulting life threatening sepsis, in her book *I Am Not Your Baby Mother*. This subject is also covered in depth by Dr Annabel Sowemimo in *Divided* and Dr Layal Liverpool in *Systemic*.

According to the most recent data, the gulf in outcomes in the UK has reduced, but mortality in black women remains elevated at three times that of white women. Before we pat ourselves on the back for any progress, it should be noted, and then shouted, that this reduction isn't necessarily because of any improvements in the care of black women – but rather perhaps because in the stripped-out, engineless sinking vessel that is the NHS, the care for white women has simply gotten *worse*. (This is what the data suggests; there has been an overall increase in maternal mortality in recent years.) As desperate as I am to see equity for everyone, this can't be achieved by opening up oppression to all-comers.

It is unsurprising that the inequality is inherited – the children of these mothers remain more likely to become ill and die. In infancy, they are three times more likely to die than the children of white mothers, and throughout childhood as a whole, the rate remains at least double.

The root (and by extension the solutions) to this can be presented as complex – an interplay between the unfair healthcare system, social situations and cultural factors. In reality, all that needs to happen is an effort to improve baseline health, listen to women when they're pregnant, in labour and after – and to then make sure the child goes home to adequate housing and healthcare. Simple.

* * *

And then, months later, it was our turn. Excitement mingled with all the usual fears and uncertainty prospective patients face – heightened by the feeling that this was still hardly a normal time to be pregnant. I say 'our', as if this were a burden equally shared, but I of course was still allowed to drink alcohol, eat mountains of sushi or go bungee-jumping if the mood took me.

I had moved on to an infinitely more civilised job, my weeks containing a hefty chunk of non-clinical research time. A perk of this was flexi-working, and although it was paid back in evenings writing up results, it did mean I could go to every scan with Louise.

The ultra-modern maternity building was a tower of white-walled concrete and glass. It looked like the sort of modern art gallery that's used to wash oligarch oil money – the place was adorned with sculptures and pictures, figuratively representing the joys of pregnancy and motherhood.

In stark contrast to the grim utilitarianism elsewhere in London NHS hospitals, it was beautiful. This almost certainly had something to do with the world-famous research programme running alongside the NHS services. And, in many ways, the clinical resources matched the building. In what has been historically one of the more deprived pockets of London, an array of tests and interventions was on offer that would have private patients wondering why they were wasting their money.

Louise and I were in a clinic room, sitting opposite one of the legion of clinical fellows, many from Central and Eastern Europe, who had come to apprentice in the arts of scanning and foetal medicine. Each appointment we saw a different one – and often two, or even three at a time, as they compared notes on the finer points of drawing measurement lines over the precious grey pixelated dots on the screen.

'What do you do for work? . . . Are you a mathematician?'

There was suspicion in her Polish-accented voice. Whenever a doctor asks you what you do in this tone, it's often because you've wrongfooted them, displaying just that little bit too much information to be a civilian. In this case, I had pushed back more than she was used to on the statistics she had presented.

'I'm a doctor . . . but I also do research.'

She smiled, but the sweetness in her expression was blended, sharpened with rictus notes.

'Okay great – so we can go over it in more detail.'

Clearly she was *thrilled* at this prospect – who doesn't love being second-guessed at work? We were weighing up our choice between two very different options, after the combined 12-week scan had placed us in a 'higher probability' category of there being a problem with the pregnancy. At the first appointment, the hokey-cokey of residual COVID restrictions had meant that, after the screening scan, I was sent back downstairs, only to return if there was an issue.

With this information, receiving a phone call in the lobby, instead of Louise stepping off the lift, had been an unwelcome warning shot.

'Matt . . . can you come back up?'

Ascending, the elevator accentuated the feeling of my legs being about to give way underneath.

It was a choice between the in-no-way-chill-sounding chorionic villus sampling – a test considered as being 'diagnostic', but also invasive, carrying the small but real risk of miscarriage, and a blood test – which doesn't, but was pitched as being less accurate, without a clear explanation of in exactly what way.

Scheduling meant we had been given the chance to go home for a few days and think about the procedure. This allowed us to firstly stew, but more importantly (in between shared crying sessions in the car), break out Google and a calculator.

I took this task on – not because I'm intrinsically more able (we had both yawned through the same medical school statistics lectures), but because it's a major part of my current job, and as I say, just like the growing a baby and dietary restrictions, the anxieties of pregnancy were never going to be shared equally. Louise's mind was on other things.

Back in the room with the obstetrician, like a politician on *Question Time* on the attack, I wheeled out my figures.

'Depending on the data you look at . . . even with the previous screening result, if we got a negative result from the blood test, this would mean a post-test probability of 0.02 per cent to 0.14 per cent . . .'

If this sounds confusing, it's because it is. I had to bring notes. Very occasionally, tedious know-it-all energy can be channelled into something useful. With a clearer idea of what a negative blood test would mean – namely the vanishingly small chance this would be a *false* negative, and *without* the possibility of causing physical harm, there wasn't really even a choice to make.

A medical degree, a job looking at data, and a chance delay in appointment availability shouldn't be necessary for you to fully understand the options being presented. I used to screw my face up when the softly spoken, experienced clinicians who took us for our 'Professional Development' modules would tell us, misty-eyed, that 'communication is the most important skill a doctor possesses'.

'Sure, Grandad, right above cutting out cancer.'

I now understand what they meant: you can do a lot of damage saying the wrong thing in the wrong way – both to patients and, less importantly, to your own career. All she had to say was: 'If you do the blood test, and it's positive, this is what it means. If you do the test and it's negative, this is what it means.' Not doing that could have had disastrous, life-changing consequences, however small the risk.

* * *

The young woman opposite wasn't the ideal roommate, if you had the choice during labour – of course, most of this wasn't her fault. Steroids for her inflammatory bowel disease had contributed to gestational diabetes during her pregnancy. This meant endless flapping around trying to set up the insulin and fluid infuser, followed by what felt like near-constant blood-glucose checking throughout the night.

In the early hours of the evening, while I was there, it was annoying – and I was reliably informed by Louise that once I had left for a luxurious eight hours in my own bed, in tandem with the pain of the induction and nausea from analgesia, it made sleeping almost impossible.

On the surface, her decision to top this all off by spending much of the night on her phone seemed a step too far – an affront to good manners and the communal spirit.

'Have you spoken to Marie? She's so two-faced . . .'

I've never understood this level of exaggerated, but ultimately petty conflict in some people's lives – all of the melodrama, the sort prompting social media posts like 'so many snakes in the grass . . . can hear them hissing'. She apparently felt the need to relay the same story at length, at high volume, to mum, then auntie, followed by another friend.

'They keep coming in and pricking my finger . . .'

Then again, labour is definitely another one of those situations when, if you can't have someone to advocate for you in person, having them at the end of the phone for moral support, and as a remote witness, is the next best thing. And if you're black, and have heard too many pregnancy horror stories from your friends and relatives, it can be essential. This is before you consider having a serious illness, as she did – one where it feels almost guaranteed an overworked SHO or midwife will make a mistake in managing, large or small, along the way.

* * *

A friend in the baby-catching business who will remain nameless had called in a favour. Finding out who the on-call obstetric team were, she knew the SpR and made sure they kept a close eye on things.

Unfortunately, nepotism is no match for NHS cuts, however – and lack of midwives meant that even after it became clear that we 'DEFINITELY WANT AN EPIDURAL', there was no way of progressing the labour and administering the drugs safely. So, we would have to wait.

When the situation finally changed, we were wheeled round to the comparative luxury of one of the solo rooms where the magic actually happens. The next wait was for the anaesthetist.

The anaesthetic registrar who eventually arrived was brisk and to the point – which was exactly what we needed.

'Now, this needle goes into the area just over your spine,' she explained, brandishing a small fencing sabre.

Louise waved her through the consenting process, happy to accept any of the complication risks – whether that be headache, bleeding or being sucked through a vortex to another dimension – to alleviate the pain.

Fortunately, the no-nonsense approach was reflected in her dexterity – and the sweet druggy relief was soon flowing. For the next few hours there was relative calm – the martyr I am, I was camped out on a makeshift cot I had constructed from a chair and a couple of spare pregnancy balls.

When it comes time to push, a clock starts – go over the limit, and the midwives and doctors get twitchy. Itchy fingers start to wander towards the ventouse and the forceps; emergency theatre space is checked. Around the two-hour mark, the midwife turned to me, with minimal urgency gestured vaguely at nothing in particular and said, 'Can you pull that, please?'

In the depths of fatigue, after a sleepless night, I was less than razor-sharp. This, combined with what I still maintain was a pretty vague instruction, meant I stared at her blankly.

'Pull the emergency buzzer!'

This shook me from my stupor, and at the klaxon, the obstetric team who had just been in minutes earlier reappeared. The consultant immediately elbowed her juniors out of the way, with a level of vigour that under different circumstances would raise an HR eyebrow.

My decision to remain as head end as possible, coupled with the modicum respect I'll reserve for privacy, mean details will be scant. Suffice to say that after some assistance and a litre of blood later, we were left with a baby and a renewed gratitude for the existence of obstetric medicine. Obviously I cried. Yet again.

* * *

The post-natal ward is more of the same – but worse. You're now forced to contend with what other neighbours and any plus-ones feel is an appropriate level of consideration.

'Praise Jesus!'

One woman clearly felt strongly that a child was a gift from God, and the only suitable show of gratitude was to watch back-to-back gospel sermons on YouTube – without headphones (the good news *is* to be shared far and wide after all). Was she going to sing along to all of the songs? *Yes*. Could she sing? *No*. Was anyone going to get her to shut up any time soon? Also *no*.

The length of time pushing meant antibiotics, and another day kept in the hospital, checking all was okay and waiting for the bloods to come back.

An improbably chirpy young SHO had taken me and the baby to the procedure room, which was up one floor, to put a cannula into her hands. Wheeling her off the ward, brand-new and strange, felt almost like stealing.

'So we just need to do a test call C . . . R . . . P . . .'

In contrast to our previous experience, she had taken her communication skills sessions to heart – and was clearly going to make sure we understood what was happening, even if it required a PowerPoint presentation or educational song to get her point across.

'This just tells us if there's any sort of infection, any inflammation.'

Dr Mittal was a chatter. An approach I'm equally prone to, she had decided to fill the awkward time spent preparing equipment with small talk.

'So, how much paternity leave will you get? What do you do?' (*Again* this question.)

'I'm actually a doctor . . . in rheumatology.'

She stopped as if pierced by an arrow, her smile momentarily fallen; in its place, a look that made clear she felt mortified.

'Oh God, I'm so sorry . . . there I was explaining CRP to you!'

'It's totally fine – I should have said sooner.'

There is no definite correct time to bring it up – too soon and there are real 'don't you know who I am' vibes. Too late, on the other hand, and it's as if you're playing secret shopper, trying to catch them out.

In an admirable performance, with far less shaky hands than if the roles had been reversed, she found what she was looking for first time. Even so, the sight of the sub-millimetre needle's bevel brutally puncturing brand-new skin was enough to make me wince.

Back down on the post-natal ward, Louise had taken the opportunity to get to the shower, which was finally free. As I sat waiting, transfixed by the now re-swaddled bundle in the Perspex box, the cycle of limited newborn states ticked back over from sleepy to 'hungry'.

Regardless of any instant, all-consuming emotions you may feel in the first days, these won't suddenly stop you being awkward in the moment. I still almost felt like needing permission as I held her tentatively, not knowing what to do with her screaming.

In the moment that I hesitated, a midwife emerged as if from nowhere and gathered her up more tightly to her chest. Even this wasn't enough, however. She clearly only wanted one thing – a swift reminder of the limits of my utility – and the howling continued until Louise returned.

CHAPTER 19

Sins of the Father

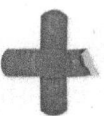

TO QUOTE JOHN F. Kennedy (via Anthony Bourdain), 'to have a child is to give fate a hostage' – and, by extension, when they are ill, in the hospital fate hands them over to strangers. This is something I couldn't fully grasp during my sole four-month paediatrics SHO job in 2014. Not that it's necessary to become a parent to empathise, to do that job well – but, for me, it has taken feeling the angst that can accompany just a sniffle, the baby clearing their throat in the night, to begin to understand parents in hospital.

As enlightened as I'd like to claim our household is, there remains a gender divide among tasks. Bins are my purview, and as I write, a fresh glistening fox shit awaits my attention in the garden, taunting me through the window, sitting atop a pile of bricks like some artefact on a plinth in the V&A. Soft furnishings, bedding, linen, on the other hand . . . sure, I'll wash them, only to have a panic attack trying to decide if something is a hand towel or a shower mat when it comes to folding them away. Parenting is another thing that can settle into a similar separation of roles if you let it, and so it was with the nights.

In the first weeks after our daughter was born, lying on the sofa in the lounge, my companions were the mercifully sleeping infant and the searing cold beam from the streetlight outside the window. The glow seemed to find my retinas wherever I lay in the room – redecorating beyond our means had meant the budget didn't extend to curtains.

This new sleeping arrangement from the hours of 11 until 2am wasn't some dog-house punishment. At least not for anything on my part, other than being 50 per cent responsible for the sleep-wrecking bundle of joy beside me – but rather because we soon realised that one bottle feed from me in the depths of the night, to allow Louise seven or so hours of unbroken rest, was what it would take to keep us away from the brink.

Thoughts of this early time induce a kind of delirious nostalgia – with the simplicity of formula, nappies and perpetual *MasterChef Australia*. Production-line parenting, the days and nights filled with endless repetitions of this limited array of tasks. In the first weeks and months, the house was a cocoon permeated by a fugue state, never fully awake or resting.

As she got older, at times getting her off to sleep could be like trying to reel in a giant marlin. Hours spent with her cradled in the rocking chair, until we washed ashore in the morning, exhausted, the bones of the night picked clean.

It's a strange cruelty that she won't remember this time of closeness with us. One of us had her at all times, knew what was happening, and what she was doing. Although this wouldn't last, at the time it all felt unending, but then suddenly was gone, the world getting bigger in steps and jolts.

It's trite to say, but when we are forced to hand over

responsibility for caring for our children, it matters who does it. The spectrum of anxiety runs from 'will nursery protect my delicate little darling from the rough kids' to whether they are going to feed my child unrefined sugar, to the possibilities of far worse. There's relief when you're sure you've found someone who will be caring and attentive, who greets your child like their own at the front door when you drop them off. But relief is accompanied by guilt when, at pickup time, the staff tell you something you didn't know about them – their new likes, their habits.

When the responsibility isn't for the (genuinely important) feeding, finger-painting and nursery rhymes, but something more serious, then the nerves and the scrutiny rachet accordingly. If your child is sick, then how well can you trust the disconcertingly young doctor in front of you to know what's wrong? Or the learned professor whose every proclamation is taken unquestioningly as gospel. Every healthcare professional who treats children has two patients – the child, and the parent, with the latter sometimes requiring more attention.

Most are trusting, grateful and reasonable – while others have legitimate concerns, highlighting things overlooked and advocating when they know their child 'just isn't themselves'. There are also those, however, for whom nothing will ever be enough to allay anxiety, fear and anger at the situation manifested as hypervigilance and mistrust. Knowing where the line is between these two is the challenge, and we must remember that the response to both needs to be understanding.

* * *

Even though, more often than not, the right care is given, mistakes are made, and overconfidence, ego and the simple, efficiently lethal truth of being too busy can intervene. The high-profile case of Martha Mills, when recounted in the blinking daylight of Radio 4's *Today* programme, made for agonising listening – not just for parents, but for any medic removed from the situation. It's hard to imagine a clearer story of a patient's descent – accompanied by the parents' urgent, unheard calls to do the right thing.

By all accounts, Martha was a lively, intelligent and, most importantly, completely healthy 13-year-old, who sustained an injury while riding her bike. She had slipped, and been struck in the abdomen by her handlebars. Rather than just the knocks kids sustain all the time falling off their bikes, she sustained a laceration to her pancreas.

What followed was a nightmare sequence of parental concerns being dismissed as their child deteriorated – starting with the doctor in the local minor injuries unit, who decided they didn't need to review her when contacted by the nurse who had seen her. It ended up with what sounds like catastrophic levels of hubris from team members at the world-renowned centre where she was eventually transferred. This led to her sepsis being undertreated and prevented them from moving her from their ward to intensive care, even after it was indicated. She died – without everything being done that was possible to prevent it. Merope Mills's retelling in the *Guardian* should be required reading for medical students and doctors.

Her parents were well-spoken, middle-class professionals – one, an editor at the aforementioned major national newspaper, someone who communicates at the highest level for a living. If they weren't listened to, in the light of concern and clinical information that in the piece sounds so clear you'd hope most medical students would get it right, then what hope does anyone else have? Subconsciously, there's nothing like Received

Pronunciation and the spectre of the Patient Advice and Liaison Service (PALS) office to keep staff on their best behaviour – but in this case that wasn't enough.

It's hard to comment on exactly what happened from the medical team's perspective – we have the account of grieving parents, and the coroner's report, the recommendations to protect future patients. I find it doubtful, but there could be some small nuance I can't see, some additional explanation, but a keen appreciation of nuance won't change the outcome.

It would be disingenuous to have protested earlier about systemic failings in the cases of ethnic minority doctors, and now suggest that one specific person is to blame. I can already hear the cry of double standards. The system failed in this instance and the hospital have made public the steps they're taking to make sure it never happens again.

Notice no one has been struck off (although one doctor has faced a tribunal without suspension), no one has been threatened with prison; instead, the focus has been on trying to fix things. This happened at a specialist hospital, but there is nothing special about the human and structural factors that contributed. This could have happened in any of the hallowed institutions in which patients place their trust.

There has also been the very visible campaign to ensure the right of patients, parents and other relatives to a second opinion when they feel escalation of care is needed. Martha's Rule, as it is known, has been rolled out – with phone numbers available allowing the concerned to contact critical care outreach staff and trigger such a review. The evidence from the institution of similar rules elsewhere (for example 'Ryan's Rule' in Australia) suggests benefit, empowering patients and, ultimately, anything that recentres those at the heart of care can only be a good thing.

We should welcome everything that helps us do a near impossible job better. Paediatrics is a wrongfooting blend of ultimately well children with temporary, common illnesses who will get better, and mercifully less common, rarer, often harrowing stories of those who won't. A generalist at a district hospital can be expected to think of and deal with anything – bronchiolitis, genetic metabolic disease, malaria. To do it well, it takes a particular temperament – the ability to transition seamlessly from an in-depth conversation with a five-year-old about *Paw Patrol* to intubating a neonate.

* * *

Since becoming a parent, it's as if a swirling, fluid ball of plasma sits in the middle of my chest. Unmoulded, shapeless emotion – it can make all other feelings appear to be a hollow effigy by comparison. But it is not always gentle. It can easily become anger, outwards at the world for not being safe enough, not being certain enough. I can now recognise and forgive even the worst interactions I have with parents in hospital, even when their concerns are unfounded, or at least misdirected.

Back in 2014, however, it was RSV season, so the ward was overrun with wheezing, gunk-streaming, miserable infants, accompanied by their desperate, sleep-deprived parents. Although potentially serious, everyone we saw would almost certainly get better, but not before they had put the adults through a couple of days of hell. Lying on camp beds next to their child, they endlessly struggled to keep the oxygen prongs on and the fluids down.

It's never a good idea to rush – so the ward round was long. The consultant, Dr Mitchell, seemingly refreshed her supply of concern anew each time – even as the stereotyped stories meant patients could start to blur. But one stood out – certainly because they weren't admitted with breathing difficulties, but also because of what *was* wrong with them.

This little girl was having a flare-up of a chronic health condition that is so rare, that at the time I had to look it up to remind myself what it was, having not encountered it other than as a footnote in a medical school lecture. It's also sufficiently uncommon that if I told you the exact disease, some simple maths could allow the parents and patient to identify themselves without much ambiguity.

When a child with one of these exotic, bird of paradise illnesses lands on the ward, it's more than even the heroically adaptable general paediatricians can be expected to manage solo. The call goes in to the specialists at the ivory tower – seeking advice on management and to ask if they fancy taking them off our hands (often the answer to the latter is a polite no – preferring instead to dish out advice from afar).

Patients with strange diseases need strange blood tests – the samples then couriered off, having to keep faith that all the correct life-saving boxes on the form have been ticked, and that they'll find their way to a mysterious lab in another part of the city. Until the results are back, there's almost no way to know how we're doing.

When we had seen her on the ward round, Mariam had been perfectly happy – although initially shy, she had been won over by the ever-reliable combination of the consultant's charm and sticker collection. She had been admitted with a UTI – which in turn had triggered a flare-up of her illness, but she was weathering it like a champ, sitting smiling on her mother's lap. As we started to make the standard self-extraction noises and movements to round off the consultation, her father, who until then had been a wall of near silence, took the opportunity to press home the importance and urgency of getting results back as soon as possible.

'Doctor, please don't forget the blood tests.'

The situation had galvanised his baseline intensity – and it punctuated his speech, which, thanks to years living in the UK, was a blend of their native West African (I am being deliberately vague here to avoid risking my GMC number) and London tones.

'Don't worry, as soon as they're back, we'll let you know.'

This was perhaps less of a reassurance than Dr Mitchell had intended to suggest. The only part of this process we had any control over was just that – relaying information once it was available. There wasn't really anything we could do to put some extra juice into the pipette arm of a lab technician in another hospital to crank them out any faster.

The round groaned on. It takes as long as it takes, and today it was just Dr Mitchell, Sam the registrar, who was regularly being pulled away to douse embers before they became fires elsewhere on the ward, and me, the SHO. A glorified scribe, I was documenting the consultations in 'please don't sue me' medical legalese, and adding to the ever-lengthening list of jobs I'd be toiling over once we were done.

Alongside the cookie-cutter discharge summaries – 'respiratory distress, wheeze . . . nebuliser . . . admitted for observation and fluids . . .' – this list included 'chasing' the bloods from St Elsewhere. The word 'chase' is contentious – now, as a slightly more grown-up doctor, almost ready to shed my shiny specialist L plates, if I'm ever reviewing a patient and I see in the referring team's plan 'chase rheumatology review', I get a twinge of professional insult. And who are *you*? Implying I need whipping to do my job. Still, as a house officer, chasing is what the plan said, so chasing is what I did.

* * *

It was gone lunchtime, and in the corridor outside the office, the girl's father had become an animated presence that couldn't be ignored. Leaving the mundane security of the discharge summary, I headed to the door like a prisoner to the gallows.

Perseverance had given way to impatience, impatience to anger – and now anger had become fury. As well as dishing out pointers on non-confrontational body language for staff to adopt, the mandatory conflict resolution training videos list indications that someone is becoming increasingly upset, and at risk of unleashing verbal or physical abuse. Presumably this is for the benefit of staff who have never found themselves in a south London pub on Friday night to witness them first hand. We were approaching a full bingo card – pacing, hands up, and baring his teeth. It was surreal watching the signs manifest and calmly ticking them off in a parallel thought track to the more pressing awareness that I could quite easily soon be punched in the face.

'How many times? I told you it's important, but you still don't have them?!'

'But there's nothing we can do – when we last checked, the lab hadn't processed them . . .'

'And when was that? You should be checking now!'

'We will, but we have lots of jobs – we do have other patients as well . . .'

This is most definitely *not* the correct thing to say – even if mathematically correct, on a ward with 20 other kids, to the parents, there is always only one patient.

This was the breaking point. The decibel level was now such that this was the only event on the ward.

'My daughter is going to have brain damage because of *you*!'

'I promise, we're trying our best.'

The conviction had evaporated from my delivery.

'It's not good enough!'

I had run out of responses and was reduced to stammering – however, Sam, the nurse in charge, chose this moment to tag himself in.

'Sir, you're going to have to go back to the room. Like he said, we can't make them do it any faster, and this isn't helping anyone.'

This was delivered with a delicate balance of calm, and the firmness of a nightclub bouncer, honed over years of shepherding the understandable, if sometimes unfairly targeted, fears of parents.

Although it didn't placate him, it did at least seem to stall the climb in his anger. Still seething, he did as he was asked and turned back to his daughter's room, shout-whispering something that sounded distinctly like 'fucking useless' as he went.

* * *

A significant body of research from the US illustrates the racial disparities in the healthcare of children, affecting both the treatment of patients, and the experience of interacting with the system for parents, at all stages in childhood and across all specialties.

For example, a review of the available literature found black and other non-white children were less likely than their white counterparts to receive adequate pain relief following a fracture, and likewise less likely to receive intravenous fluid for dehydration in cases of gastroenteritis – even when controlled for factors such as insurance. As with other similar disparities, many of the reasons underlying this will be structural – but, in particular, the pre-existing biases of staff are no doubt a major factor.

Under these circumstances, mistrust is not then necessarily misplaced – and confrontation may be an unfortunate, but appropriate, last-resort response, an attempt to ensure your child gets the care they need. However, black and other ethnic minority parents have to worry about being perceived as over-emotional or adversarial – labelled as 'difficult', or, at the other end of the spectrum, seen as insufficiently worried about the health of their child. Parents also fear they are more likely to be referred for investigation by social services, and this is borne out in the evidence.

This same issue is understudied in the UK – to the point where the absence of research is glaring. While we are clearly not just a little America, we aren't so different that we can be confident we're not replicating the same here. Given the signals from almost all other areas of healthcare, in particular pregnancy and peri-partum care, I'm confident in many ways we are alike.

Being engaged in the care of your sick child is not free. Parents with professional jobs are more likely to have a degree of flexibility, able to make up time taken to attend appointments or work remotely (still by no means an easy proposition). Many parents from ethnic minorities will clearly fall into this category, but access to this sort of work is not equal. For those working manual jobs, on the other hand, attending appointments or having a child in the hospital means risking lost income, or your job entirely.

These differences in care feed into the aforementioned worse outcomes among non-white children. Health cannot be neatly separated from the other facets of their lives – and it's likely a significant proportion of this burden is due to higher levels of deprivation. It is also likely, however, that the structures of the healthcare system itself and the attitudes and actions of staff share in the blame.

* * *

Staffroom is a generous word for the converted windowless cupboard that served that purpose on the ward. Sponge erupted from gashes in the upholstery on the chairs, and laminate peeled on every surface.

This was to be the setting of our debrief – with distinctly more interrogation cell than wellness vibes. Fortunately, Sam was far more sympathetic than the room. Sitting opposite in one of the dilapidated perches, he was genuinely keen to check I was okay, even though nothing had really happened in the end, aside from a little shouting and the suggestion we were a team of uncaring incompetents.

'Are you alright?'

'Yeah . . . I just don't know what he expects us to do . . .'

I could feel the familiar shudder that accompanied the adrenaline of a confrontation, a fight at school win or lose, sending ripples through my words. Worse, I could feel the sting of tears (fourth time in this book if you're counting) and desperately sought to somehow expand and contort my eyelids to contain them. Regardless of how progressive a world we think we now live in, we're not well equipped to deal with men crying, unless they're crying big, muscular, manly tears celebrating a sporting triumph. There's no way around it – it's just awkward.

I managed to avert a full-blown lachrymose breakdown. Sensing it would be best for all involved if I took a minute, Sam got up and headed back to the ward to deal with the thousand other things that had momentarily been set aside in favour of this spectacle.

When I emerged a few minutes later, the father was waiting again, but entirely changed. Seemingly gone was the rage, replaced by the contrition and regret of letting his temper control him, anger's hangover. Arms open and smiling almost manically, he walked forward.

'My brother, I'm sorry.'

Although this sudden appeal to his version of our shared solidarity came out of left field, it was infinitely preferable to the alternative.

'It's fine,' I lied.

He continued his advance, and he put one arm round me in the gregarious embrace of the man on a night out who's had one too many, and is now meandering along the fine line between bonhomie and violence.

'In fact, why don't I go and call the lab again to see if there's any update on the test.'

I used this familiar old excuse to wriggle free and retreat to the relative safety of the office. When we finally got the result, mid-afternoon, the levels of the unspecified blood test were fine, in what now feels like the inevitable outcome. The data was relayed by the lab technician in a bored voice, divorced from the drama that the wait had caused.

Needless to confirm, I didn't become a paediatrician. Thanks in no small part to the granite-jawed but gentle ER heroism of George Clooney's Dr Doug Ross, many hopefuls (me) ended up with a skewed vision of the specialty. The fact that you want to do medicine and feel like you get on well with kids isn't enough. You have to deal with them not just when they're fun, but when they're sick and upset. You have to traumatise them with blood tests that no one in the room (you included) wants to happen. And if you don't get it quite right, you'll have to explain yourself to their parents.

Epilogue

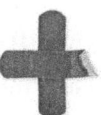

OTHER SPECIALTIES PROBABLY don't believe we have emergencies in rheumatology. They think that, when not in clinic, we retreat to the office for tea and contemplation. The amount of time I spend in A&E might contest this, however.

From colleagues' notes, at times there is a barely concealed meaning between the lines, peeking out like a silhouetted figure at the window behind the blinds. She had picked up the unwritten label of 'challenging' – again, something that seems to have a disproportionate tendency to stick to black patients (suspicion of this bias is borne out in research).

Now in her mid-thirties, but diagnosed aged 16, when she was still at school, she had the misfortune of receiving the one-two punch of lupus and rheumatoid arthritis simultaneously (a combination sometimes given the misleadingly cutesy name 'rhupus'). Suddenly she was in pain, her hair was falling out and she had rashes scarring her face. Being diagnosed young meant there had been plenty of time to fall out with her doctors.

Either of these diagnoses, at any age, is life-changing. At a time when you're supposed to be enjoying, and perhaps misusing, your growing independence, to be told you have 'arthritis', something your nan suffers from, can send you off the rails. In my experience, teenagers and young adults want to wake up remembering (often barely) the fun they had last night; they don't want to start their days, joints creaking, reaching for a cup of pills.

This is a well-recognised issue in treating young patients with chronic illnesses. Rebellion can take the self-destructive route of what is diplomatically referred to as 'non-concordance' – not taking their medication. If we're not careful, this can set up an odd dynamic: get the lecturing wrong, and patients think they're taking it for your benefit, not theirs. They feel the need to lie to you in order to keep you happy.

There is a feeling among doctors treating lupus that many patients aren't taking most of the things listed at the top of their clinic letters. This is understandable; a lot of what we prescribe can cause unpleasant side effects – as they are, in a way, as one consultant used to remind us, 'poisons used in just the right amounts'. A quick google, and the less trusting patients would think the worst about our intentions.

Another unfortunate truth is that not all of the drugs work for all people. The more of these they cycle through at a young age, with persistent symptoms still breaking through, the more they will conclude they may as well not bother. This conspires with all of the other factors which, hopefully by now, I have convinced you can dent the relationship between black patients and their doctors.

Clara fulfilled all of the above – getting her to take medications had been a battle, and even when she had, they weren't up to the task, and her symptoms had gradually gotten worse. Now she was sitting in the emergency department, because the pain in her ankles was too much. I activated the concierge routine.

'I'm Matt, one of the rheumatology doctors. Do you want to come with me?'

'Sure.'

Although the response was monosyllabic, it was better than it could have been, said with a guarded smile, so I counted myself lucky. On this occasion, her scalp had been spared by the worst of the flare-up and what seemed to be her own hair was twisted into small Bantu knots. She was sitting in a hospital wheelchair – the kind that is built for longevity and stability, not manoeuvrability. The handling is so bad, it's difficult to push without clearing half the waiting room, sending chairs and patients scattering. Still, I managed to get her to the consultation room without injuring her further.

'Okay, they said on the phone your ankles are the problem. Can I have a look, please?'

'The last doctor who did this messed me up, like he couldn't wait to be done – had me screaming.'

'Okay, well, I'll aim to avoid that then – but I'm pretty confident I'll be able to do this.'

'Pretty confident?'

'Okay, *very* confident.'

'If you say so. Also, I don't like needles.'

Much like hospitals, the proportion of people who actually *like* needles is very low – but needle phobia is most definitely a thing, particularly among those whose formative years have been punctuated by them.

These details are often disregarded, however. We seem committed to meanness, particularly as soon as patients transition into adult services (aged 16 or 18, depending on where you work).

Gone are the long appointments, games in the waiting areas and extra consideration given to not traumatising them. Sudden confrontation with the 'suck it up and get on with it' attitude of the adult world can be destabilising, and further damages the relationship.

Both of her ankles were swollen; below the shin they looked like small water balloons. With that much fluid, the procedure should have been easy, but long-suffering joints in inflammatory arthritis can deceive – the ultra-slow-motion car crash of inflammation leaves them damaged, the joint space caged in a nest of bone spurs. Any attempt with a needle is met with crunching, grimacing resistance.

I didn't say any of this, however, and instead went about the ritualistic, compulsive process of laying out the equipment for the procedure. Knowing she would only give me one chance, I took the necessary time to prepare.

Making a small, circular indentation on the skin, I reassured her: 'Don't worry, this is just me marking the area. I'll tell you when I'm doing anything with the needle.'

'You'd better.' The tone was of jovial menace.

After a blast of anaesthetic spray, we were ready.

'Okay, I'm going to do it now.'

The needle slid perfectly, unimpeded, into position – and the comically large syringe started to fill almost immediately with amber fluid, then the steroids went in. The second ankle was equally straightforward, and at this point, I knew I was on safe ground. The contrast between this and the alleged torture she had previously been put through had apparently nudged me into her good graces.

The remainder of our time was spent talking about anything other than medicine. When she was well, she worked in fashion –

but her health meant that the gaps between jobs were getting longer. Working freelance, for as many hours as the task takes, often standing on screaming feet, isn't compatible with arthritis that's out of control.

I will be a consultant soon. So much of that progression is about the synthesis of the medicine with everything else – recognising who may need some extra time, and a more oblique approach. Understanding the other factors that might come to bear on a consultation, the patient's experience of being in the world, how they are treated. Whenever I'd receive these pearls from some veteran as a medical student, I'd roll my eyes. It sounded like so much pretentious self-aggrandisement.

I am under no illusion that in a single consultation I have managed to repair her relationship with the speciality. Or that because of some magic insight on my part, and the fact I happen to look a little more like her family and friends, she will now diligently take all of her medications.

Nor am I delusional enough to think I have gotten it right every time – or ever will. I'm sure there are many patients out there less enamoured with my abilities, who will have found me smug, rude, or just not their cup of tea. But it is these encounters that serve as a metre for your development – a rare moment to acknowledge you have acquired a valuable set of skills and are the specific person who can make a patient better, even if just for today.

* * *

Perhaps I'm imagining it, but often strangers are disproport-ionately nice to men doing the most basic duty of looking after their infant children – whether it's theatrical smiling deference from the woman leaping out of the way of the pram, or a fist bump from the local eccentric street celebrity, taking a break from cheering on commuters running for the train.

As I descend the hill, pushing on into Catford proper, the parakeets' chirps blend with the pigeon coos, as the 'native' birds peck indiscriminately at the remnant scraps in takeaway boxes. But all sound is ultimately dominated by the thunder of the South Circular road. In the first year, other parents in the antenatal class obsessed about taking their babies to sensory classes, but they'd struggle to match this – the cars and sirens reaching the point of overload.

The centre is a place that, despite development, seems resistant to wholescale gentrification, for now at least. There is a shared eco system, the loud, chest-rattling bass from a reggae sound system serenades the smokers outside the windowless, resolutely non-gastro, non-chain pub, their sun-deprived skin almost translucent in the light.

Two young black men play a game of Magic: The Gathering over flat whites outside a cafe – an act of unthinkable nerdiness that, around here, would have risked an absolute pummelling when I was growing up. Meanwhile, south London's answer to those Dalston elders kiss their teeth and shake their heads at the Afghan shopkeeper's plantain prices. Cartoonishly large bottles of vegetable oil are trundled home, as mothers skilfully wrangle three times the number of children I'm contending with.

I have huge amounts of love for the place, but it's somewhere you can see life wearing on people. Every one of them could be patients in my clinic, or wheeled through on the take. Pollution, diabetes, the physical strain of a manual job, and the impossible-to-quantify burden of a life less privileged.

None of these ills are the exclusive preserve of non-white communities. There are plenty of definitely white, definitely not privileged residents of this borough. And, conversely, there are many perfectly comfortable, secure black people – overall they are in the majority. But the strain on minority communities as a whole is unequal: 34 per cent of black Londoners are defined as living in poverty, as compared to 17 per cent of their white counterparts. Even those who are financially and professionally successful are still exposed to the stresses of racialisation – this is borne out in the treatment and the outcomes I have described in these pages.

Improving the health of all such communities starts just there – in the community. A lot is being said about a shift to prevention in healthcare, away from the current model of attempting to put out the fire long after it has started. To avoid this being just buzzwords, we not only need to acknowledge the causes of people's illnesses, we must support them in making changes.

If we tell someone to eat more healthily, will we then give them access to fresh fruit and vegetables at a price that's competitive with that current demon, ultra-processed food? And, even then, will they have the time to cook? When they are doing shift work, including nights, will we encourage employers to offer staff something other than the metabolic hand grenades employees are used to? The sole offering of microwavable cheese toasties at my current hospital on a Saturday would suggest not.

We say to exercise three to four times per week, but again, when? Are patients supposed to wake up an hour early to try to fit it in before their commute, or perhaps rush to the gym before cooking that aforementioned ultra-nutritious meal? Being time-poor is not unique to minority communities, but most of the things we ask of these patients to improve their health would certainly require them becoming time-rich, cash-rich, or both.

Unfortunately, among the most important things that need to

change are the most amorphous and intangible. It's more difficult to remain well, to value your own health, when you yourself don't feel valued. The stress and low mood that can accompany living in a society that you believe isn't *for* you will manifest in your body. Correcting this would mean fundamentally altering the relationship between the structures in this country and its non-white communities.

Although by no means solved, it is possible to be optimistic about some change. In recent years, non-white people have occupied among the most senior positions in the country. To only be able to time travel, and tell Winston Churchill that the leader of the Conservative party would be a black woman, the immediate successor to a man of Indian descent, who had also served as prime minister – he'd probably need to double his famous breakfast booze order (several whisky sodas) just to steady himself. This has to be recognised for the progress it is, but it cannot be mistaken for a genuine change in the fabric of institutions that still feel constructed to favour their privileged constituencies.

One thing that almost certainly won't make the difference in isolation, and probably shouldn't in any case, is the voice of one representative like myself – someone sufficiently privileged as to be spared many, if not all, of these drains on health. What *is* needed is to speak to the people in these communities, ask them what matters to them, and what they feel will make their lives better.

* * *

When it comes to non-white staff in the NHS, some of what will improve their lives is unique, but a great deal more is the same as is needed for everyone – mainly to treat them as if they matter.

They repeatedly report experiencing discrimination, and higher rates of harassment and bullying when surveyed, as compared to their white colleagues. They also feel less likely to be considered for promotions and the opportunity to undergo training that might advance their career. While these are subjective, they can't be ignored. And across roles and professions, non-white staff remain more likely to face disciplinary proceedings and be referred to their regulator.

Some of these issues could be addressed by providing more secure means of raising concerns. As it stands, complaining about discrimination by bosses to other bosses feels like calling the police to report police brutality. The processes around promotion and training opportunities can be made less ripe for favouritism – by making them more transparent, and preventing the nurturing of managers' preferred candidate at the expense of other equally qualified staff.

Regarding medics, the GMC has at least recently acknowledged there is a problem – that non-white doctors are being over-referred. We will have to wait to see what they do about it. They certainly have the power to take this into account during the proceedings, to consider whether the person in front of them is there as much on the basis of their ethnicity as their practice.

There is less the GMC can do about the referrers and their biases – and, currently, non-medic hospital managers (who are often responsible for said referral, particularly in the case of whistleblowers) are not regulated themselves. Should this change, however, the threat of sanction, dismissal or worse might make some of them think twice before engaging in unwarranted, even vexatious referrals.

In the case of the workforce makeup, healthcare is among the most diverse industries. The ranks of doctors are a Reform voter's worst nightmare, with immigrant membership far outstripping the general population. This masks the fact that senior medical leadership, and the learned professorial ranks, are still overwhelmingly white – affecting the perceived value of non-white doctors, placing limitations on ambition. It is an oversimplification and a cliche, but we are more likely to aspire to a position when we can see ourselves in it.

The solutions offered to correct inequality inevitably end up being imperfect, often inelegant. Programmes designed to accelerate career development to make minority staff more competitive, and quotas at any stage in the hiring process, carry the stigma of positive discrimination. While they may improve diversity, they can serve to undermine successful candidates before they even start in a job. As I write, in the US in particular, DEI is suffering an existential crisis.

With diverse management and executive hiring, there is also the issue of the 'Glass Cliff' (more commonly associated with women in positions of leadership) – members of underrepresented groups only being handed the keys to a failing organisation just before the bus careers off the edge. In the process, their careers take the fall, and unfortunately, because they can never just be representing themselves, critics take this as a sage lesson about the risk of the 'diversity hire'.

If anything, the more difficult problem to address is the mismatch between aptitude and experience. Placing disadvantaged people in positions of leadership is contingent on them having acquired the skills needed to do the job – which means creating career development pipelines and access to mentorship throughout the length of careers. In an industry that requires near-constant relocation, this is no easy feat, especially when support for allocating resources to this sort of endeavour is always going to be partisan. But that shouldn't be an excuse for defeatism – this sort of help and guidance, if genuinely offered, without being patronising, will more often than not be welcomed.

* * *

None of the problems I have described, or their solutions, exist in a vacuum. Dealing with them will take place (I hope) within the NHS – assuming it continues to exist in a meaningful sense. As many who have tried accessing care in the past few years will be able to attest, this does not feel guaranteed. Whether you work in it, or are receiving treatment, it can often seem as if the sallow, grey-suited humanoids who have ultimate control over our healthcare – how it is resourced, funded and looked after – don't care about us.

The NHS may continue to remain in name, but more and more I'm coming round to agree with the more pessimistic among my colleagues – that our system is being allowed to rot from the inside. All that will be left is the external husk, with none of the core functions left to serve those who rely on it. I have heard predictions of the death of the NHS since before I started working in it. This is the first time I have genuinely worried they're not just the 'end is nigh' ravings of sandwich-board-clad doomsayers. This decline is not inevitable, however.

The NHS functions because of an unwritten, spit pact of a contract with a dedicated and knowledgeable workforce. That they will work harder, for less money than they could earn elsewhere – and, in exchange, they will be allowed to do something good, meaningful and with security. It is unhelpful to, when it suits us, label NHS staff heroes – rewarding them with doorstep claps, the echoes now long faded. It ignores the fact that they are ultimately people doing a job, with red lines in terms of pay and conditions that, once crossed, will drive them away. We are being asked to do more with less – and accept being rewarded less for the privilege.

It would be tone deaf to suggest that everyone is in the same boat – there has always been disparity and inequality between the various professions in healthcare. But at every level, that contract is being broken. Nurses and, reportedly in a few cases, out-of-work locum GPs have been forced to use food banks – this fact alone is unforgivable.

In the rush to cut costs, there is an obsession with replacing GPs in particular with allied healthcare professionals including pharmacists, paramedics and physician associates. A huge amount of digital blood has been spilled around this issue on Twitter and Reddit. I am not in the camp who feel there is no role for physician associates performing appropriate tasks, with adequate supervision in healthcare. And while, clearly, patient safety trumps DEI (although I would argue they can also often be linked), given the barriers to entering medicine, it is difficult to disentangle the debate from inequalities in class and educational opportunity.

I have worked with one experienced physician associate in acute medicine who, when she is at work, performing a role for which she is trained, makes the ward run infinitely more smoothly – like the expeditor at a peak-time restaurant. But there have been instances of salaried GPs being made redundant, because it was more economical to replace them with non-medics – and be under no illusion, the skill sets are not the same, and this risks harm. There is real appetite to prevent access to something simple that is generally considered to work as long as it's funded – namely being able to see a doctor when you need to, ideally one who knows you.

There is also the belief that AI may be about to come

along and save healthcare – ChatGPT in a white coat will be diagnosing your problems, reading your scans and holding your hand while it breaks the bad news. While it's clear there are many tasks AI can do already, such as analysing images, I'll start to fear for my job when it can sort out something as simple, but soul-crushingly time-consuming, as the mountain of admin generated every time I go near a patient.

Of course there are inefficiencies in our system, and spending money indiscriminately, without clear strategy and objectives, won't change things. I know this. I have been working here for 12 years; I have waded through and nearly drowned in the treacle. But don't believe anyone when they tell you that there is a clever AI solution to the fact you can't get an appointment, or you've waited 18 months for an operation. Until we have access to a fully functioning army of Robodocs, the answer is paying someone to sit in a room, listen to you, make a diagnosis – and then giving them the resources to treat it. Refusal to invest in paying for services adequately is rendering GPs and hospitals unable to deliver the care people expect.

Most doctors care deeply about being able to provide care, free at the point of need. If you jeopardise our futures, however, we will turn elsewhere, and it is already happening. Private GPs used to be the preserve of a rarefied few, the type for whom Waitrose is a little déclassée. Now, with primary care seemingly on life support, it's become normalised for anyone desperate not to wait a month for an appointment. On escalators on the tube, on social media, I'm greeted by the warm vicarly smiles of the transaction medic, advertising their services – there in an instant if you have the readies.

Doctors can be divided into thirds. There are those among us who were already committed to the *business* of medicine. At the other end of the spectrum, the idealists would fall on their scalpels rather than demand cash from their patients before care. In the middle is a group who are happy to serve the people via the NHS exclusively, up until their mortgages are threatened, or the system dumps on them one time too many. There are only so many times they will accept turning up to work to find they are seeing twice as many patients, doubling their risk, for less money. I now speak to GPs who in the past would never have dreamed of working outside the NHS, who are now scrabbling to understand the bureaucracies of CQC registration and self-marketing.

The plight and financial woes of senior medics, who are undoubtedly overall well paid relative to the population, may not even be worth breaking the tiny violin from its case. Whether they keep showing up to work in the NHS should matter to you, however. If there is an exodus to private practice, it goes without saying that the results will be unjust. There is a two-tier health service on the horizon, with inequalities eclipsing the stratification that already exists. Those who can't afford to flee and follow their doctors will be left to survive among the ruins – waiting, living with pain for longer, and dying sooner.

This shift is also likely to disadvantage some minority ethnic and non-male staff – as preferences and prejudices become market forces. When paying for an opinion, patients will seek a learned source who matches their expectations. This will often be someone male, over 45, of the same ethnicity – which, based on who is more likely to be able to afford it, means white.

I am also firmly of the belief that there are still a huge number of things that the NHS does better, and most importantly more safely than the private hospitals. In many cases it is still apparent that the warm lighting, Egyptian cotton bedding and monogrammed towels are at the expense of functioning emergency response teams and procedures. When things fall apart, private hospitals are still offloading patients to the local A&E to put them back together. This may not be the case forever, as providers eye up the limping prey and seek to provide more comprehensive services all under one roof – following the model that, funnily enough, again, seems to work pretty well if you fund it . . .

Ironically, given the likely greater barrier to access, patients from minority groups might have the most to gain from seeing a private doctor in their clinic. If they were viewed as paying customers, they may be greeted more pleasantly, listened to more attentively. If there is one thing the public sector could learn from the private sector, it is to stop treating patients like an inconvenience.

This is an echo of the sentiment expressed in *I Am Not Your Baby Mother*, as she weighed up sending her child to private school. Regardless of any hangups there may be, when the institution providing a service wants your money, and recognises that the easiest way they can get it is by doing the best for you, regardless of your skin colour, that is what they will do.

This doesn't need to be the final word – the decision to let the NHS drift towards oblivion is just that: a choice. There is nothing other than the will to do it preventing us from demanding that resources are allocated to at least doing the basics well. Train enough doctors, and then pay GP practices a viable amount of money to employ them to provide appointments. This is a simple supply and demand problem, with a straightforward solution. Healthcare that is free in your time of need, regardless of your circumstances, is precious. To lose it would be to betray the best part of ourselves.

Acknowledgements

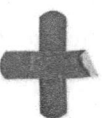

I'll have to begin with an apology – it's almost impossible to adequately thank everyone who played a role in bringing this book to life. This process has shown me how in many ways, it's farcical that only the author's name makes it on to the cover. I owe gratitude to everyone close to me who has allowed me to include their story in this book.

First, thanks to my wife 'Louise'. Thank you for encouraging and supporting me through a process that has often turned precious time away from the hospital and the lab into yet another workday – and for putting up with all of this landing in the same year as the other small task of my PhD write-up. You have the patience of a particularly put-upon saint.

Thanks too to my children, for showing me what's important – whether by smiling, laughing or keeping me awake through the night.

To my parents – anyone who has read this far will understand the role you played in creating an environment that has allowed me to pursue a career in medicine and beyond. What they won't have seen, however, are the countless other things you do for us that have made writing this book possible. Paying back the free childcare alone would bankrupt us.

To my brother – for being the other side of so many nonsensical conversations over the years growing up, which no doubt have formed the bases for my 'comedy' – and for being honest when any creative endeavour I show you 'needs a bit more work'.

To Alf – for being the loudest cheerleader – bragging to half of Birmingham long before we'd really achieved anything at all.

Thanks to Louise's family – for many things, but in particular, for allowing me to share 'Edward's' story, and to him for being an amazing father, grandfather and father-in-law.

Thanks to my friends – especially those who have allowed me to include them in the book – Tommy, Ryan, Kyron, Joel, Ruari and 'Josh'. Your cavalier disregard for your own privacy is admirable. I also owe thanks to Benji Waterhouse – who having been through the whole publishing process before me, has been an invaluable source of advice and motivation.

To Rowan Lawton, my agent at the Soho Agency and Julian Alexander – thanks for your indispensable help taking the barely formed idea I brought to you, moulding it into a proposal and then continuing to push until the finish. Thanks also to Helen Mumby, for helping the book find its way to into the hands of people who may help give the book another life beyond print.

To everyone at Bonnier Books who has worked on the book, this really has been a collaboration – Rik Ubhi for taking a chance and giving the book a home, editor Matt James for reining in authorial indulgences and excesses and bringing clarity – as well as Ciara Lloyd, James Lilford and Madiya Altaf for the finishing touches. Thanks also to Victoria Denne for copyediting and Ross Jamieson for proof reading. To Alex Kirby, thanks for delivering to me a career first – graphic design that perfectly captured everything I wanted, first time. Thanks to Clare Kelly and Sophie Raoufi for pushing the book, getting it in front of people and making sure it will actually be read. Thanks to Charlotte Brown at Bonnier, Lucy Wroe and the team at Small Wardour for your work on the audiobook – and making three days listening to the sound of my own voice in a booth an enjoyable experience.

Thanks to the NHS colleagues, and of course the patients with whom I have shared the experiences, good and bad, that formed these stories. Hopefully I have done you justice.

Last of all, thanks to you, reader, for picking this book up and making it to the end – without you, this might as well all have remained an unrealised dream.